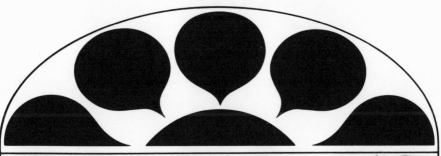

A GUIDE TO NATURAL

COSMETICS

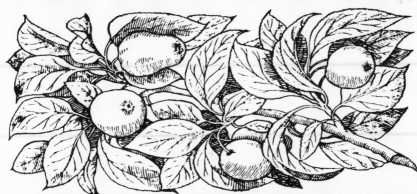

CONNIE KROCHMAL

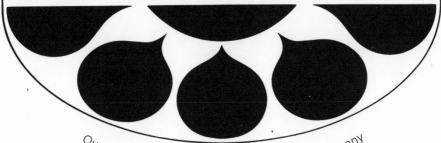

Quadrangle/The New York Times Book Company

Library of Congress Catalog Card Number: 73-77028
International Standard Book Number: 0-8129-0362-5

Production by Planned Production
Designed by Hermann Strohbach

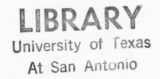

ACKNOWLEDGMENTS

I am much indebted to Emanuel Geltman, Editor, Quadrangle Books, for his encouragement and support to me in writing this book; to Dr. I. T. Littleton, Director of the D. H. Hill Library, North Carolina State University, and his efficient staff for their never-failing willingness to help locate information and sources of information; to my husband's Cornell classmate, Dr. W. Grierson, and his colleagues Jim Kesterson, C. D. Atkins, and Dr. W. F. Wardowski, of the Institute of Food and Agricultural Sciences, University of Florida, Lake Alfred, for providing experimental samples of various citrus oils and essences; to our family druggist, R. I. Cromley, R.Ph., of Cromley's Pharmacy, Raleigh, North Carolina, for his patience and cooperation in finding sources of information as well as for his ideas and comments.

The illustrations were generously provided by Dr. Earl Core, Biology Department, University of West Virginia; L. R. Newby, Director, Department of Information and Extension Service, Government of Papua and New Guinea; Edward Telesford, of the British Museum; the American Spice Trade Association; and *France Actuelle*.

Raleigh, North Carolina   C.K.

CONTENTS

A GUIDE TO
NATURAL
COSMETICS

Introduction

COSMETICS—WHAT ARE THEY?

⌈The word "cosmetic" came to us from the ancient Greeks, whose word *kosmein* meant "to decorate." Cosmetics in our society have a wide range of meanings, all basically referring to a means of making a person more attractive by whatever contemporary standards are in vogue.⌉

Although we think of "cosmetic" as a term applied to things put on the face, hair, arms, and other parts of the body, the term "cosmetic surgery" refers to such applications as the remodeling of noses, the repair of scars and unsightly blemishes, and the once fashionable operation called face lifting. Cosmetic surgery, in fact, has been used for centuries. For example, flat heads were considered desirable in some early societies such as the Flathead Indians of our own United States, and children had their heads flattened. In parts of Africa, a broad lower lip was considered attractive, and the Ubangi inserted a small wooden disc into the lower lip to make the wearer attractive. Then, too, tattooing has been considered a fashionable form of decoration by a number of peoples. It was known and practiced by the ancient Egyptians and the early residents of Britain; and present-day Papuans and Tahitians, among others, also admire tattooed designs on the skin.

I shall not consider these practices in this book because they are not used in modern households. Rather, I shall consider those methods of enhancing attractiveness and appearance that are within the realm of practicality in the ordinary American home.

⌈Primitive people, mostly men, used face and body cosmetics to protect themselves from evil—and to record their brave deeds in battle. In part, the use of decorative cosmetics on men's faces and bodies was sexually oriented, an effort to make the wearer more attractive to the females of the groups. Both men and women painted the face and body, as well as the hair—and still do today in certain parts of the world—to announce some spiritual crisis: war, death, marriage, and

1

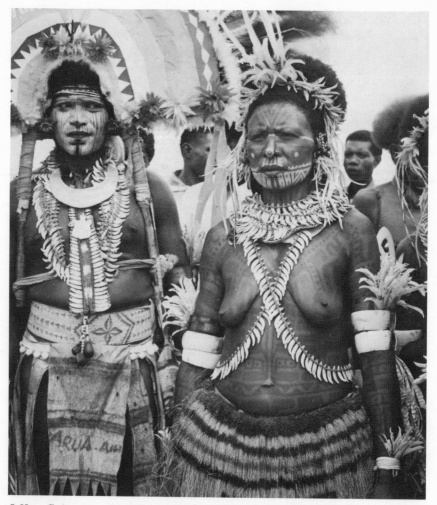

A New Guinea couple of the central coastal district, tattooed and painted in formal and ceremonial fashion. Department of Information, Territory of Papua and New Guinea.

sometimes the birth of a child. The Maoris of New Zealand, the Papuans and New Guineans, and many African people still decorate their bodies and faces for special events. Body paints were also used for identification, as tribal units became more and more a part of the human scene. Some body decorations were used as a means of fooling evil spirits and djinns. To this day in some lands a baby boy is given a gold ring to wear to make the Evil Ones believe he is a girl. (Apparently girls are far less desirable to them than are little boys.) I myself wear such a ring, one that my husband wore when he was a baby.

THE COSMETICS OF ANCIENTS

Among the early Jews, the Babylonian Talmud clearly required a husband to provide his wife with cosmetics, partly for attractiveness but equally for cleanliness. The Hebrews' preoccupation with sanitation and body cleanliness set them apart from their contemporary neighbors. Moses clearly and unmistakably ordered his people to guard their bodies as being a gift of God—an attitude shared by the Greeks and Romans, who concurred in the Jewish belief that the body was a temple and an object of respect.

(Some cosmetics began to be used because of a real need. Archaeologists have found that the people who settled in Egypt, the ancestors of the ancient Egyptians, used the oil of the castor bean plant as a protection against the burning rays of the desert sun.] Their descendents, the Egyptians of history, continued to use castor oil for the same

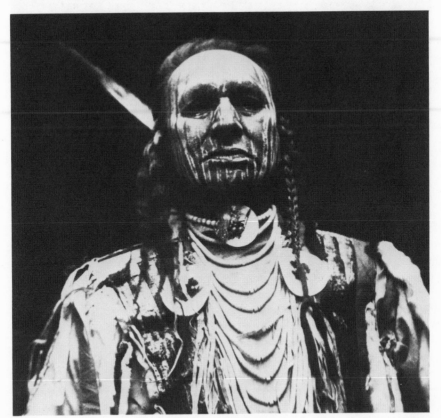

This old photo shows Mars-che-coodo, or "White Man Runs Him," a Crow scout for General Custer, adorned with ceremonial painting. Smithsonian Institution, National Anthropological Archives, Negative No. 3409-b.

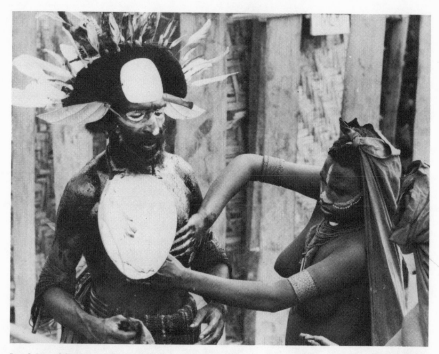

Lard is rubbed on visitors to the Mount Hagen district in the western highlands of New Guinea. This social gesture of welcome is not only considered decorative, but it helps keep the body warm at chilly highland temperatures. Department of Information, Territory of Papua and New Guinea.

purpose. They learned to protect their eyes from the sun's glare by applying a green copper compound, as paintings in ancient tombs reveal; thus they developed a beautifying cosmetic to meet a common need.

In the New Guinea highlands the age-old custom of greeting guests by rubbing them with lard is still carried on. This social gesture arose from a host's concern that his guest should not suffer from the low temperatures common in the mountains. Lard helps maintain body warmth at a comfortable level.

Hair decoration was highly important to the Egyptians, a mode probably borrowed from the Assyrians, who spent incredibly long hours shaping and preening their hair and, in the case of men, their long and luxuriant beards. Oils and unguents were used, and in the society of those days hair styles were tied very much to status and rank. I am fairly sure that the farmer or laborer and his wives had little time for the elaborate hairdressing of the upper class.

Perfumes are believed to have been first used in Egypt, by priests preparing mummified bodies for interment. Egyptian tombs have been found with elaborate toilet kits in them, giving us some idea of the cosmetic tools and supplies used in those days.

The Romans, originally a virile and masculine group, respected their bodies and believed in properly caring for them, through baths and exercise. However, as they conquered their neighbors in several directions, they picked up habits that were not in keeping with their early martial simplicity. They began to frequent massage parlors where highly scented body oils were used, usually by attractive slaves of either sex. From Germany they brought back the custom of using hair grease made from the scented fat of some animal. Some of them spread a white lead powder over their faces—a dangerous practice that, then and now, can lead to death.

In the wonderful old city of Pompeii, destroyed in 79 A.D. by an eruption of the volcano Vesuvius, archaeologists have found the remains of an old soap factory. It is interesting to speculate that the Roman legions occupying the land of the Germans noted that the tribesmen used a soap made of animal fats and ashes, copied the method, and brought it back to Rome, from where it spread to other parts of Italy.

The ancient Greeks were remarkably advanced in health and sanitation; public baths and public toilets were common in the city-states.

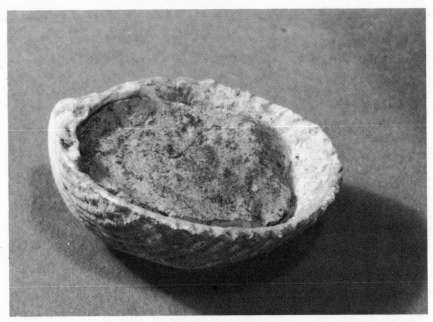

From the ruins of ancient Ur came this sea-shell beauty aid. In it is malachite, a green mineral material used in ancient times as a form of eye "shadow" for protection from the burning sun. Trustees, British Museum, London.

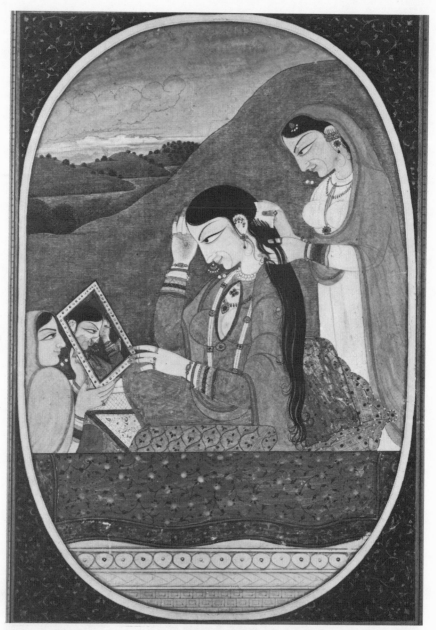

This painting "Lady with a mirror" represents the use of cosmetics and make-up by women of India. Victoria and Albert Museum, London.

A typical public toilet had stone seats, built over a flowing stream. However, the Greeks in general were so strongly trained for a life of service to the state, military discipline, and the value of being an athlete that few cosmetics were used—other than by the local prostitutes who made use of various cosmetic materials to clearly denote their trade.

The early inhabitants of England painted themselves blue with a plant called woad, both for attractiveness and to mark social events; and some Eskimos still use a blue color as a facial ornament.

On the Indian subcontinent women were long ago encouraged to use perfumes, bath oils, breath sweeteners, and whatever cosmetics their imaginations led them to believe would enhance their attractiveness to their husbands. The famed Indian love manuals, the *Kama Sutra* and *The Perfumed Garden*, tell of some of the cosmetics used, and the consequences.

With the sack of Rome by barbarian hordes and the end of the Roman empire of the Caesars, bathing and cosmetics disappeared from Europe, remaining out of view, and smell, for several centuries.

COSMETICS IN THE DARK AGES

In about the eighth century, soap reappeared in Italy, and found its way to France by the thirteenth century. Soap was made in England in the early 1600s, but the government, in stern disapproval of such

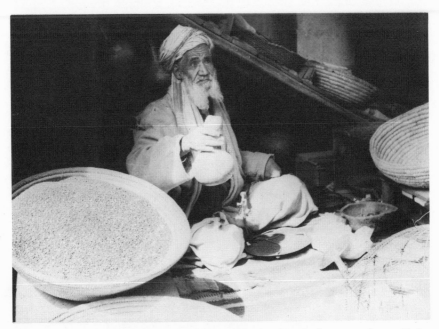

This handsome Afghan patriarch in Kabul sells dried herbs for aromatic use in the home as well as medicinal herbs that are much in demand. Arnold Krochmal.

foreign fripperies, taxed the product heavily to discourage sturdy yeomen from becoming effeminate, like the continentals.

As Christianity moved west from the Holy Land, it brought with it some new concepts, differing from the Jewish, Roman, and Greek respect for the body. The early Christians did not feel that to be holy required one to be dirty, nor that to be dirty meant that one was holy. But they did feel that the body was a more or less temporary receptacle for a soul intended for higher duties, and that overconcern with the body could perhaps lead to spiritual problems. Eventually the Puritan ethic carried this further by suggesting that the body was a dormant source of evil and that pampering something with such a potential for sin was much to be decried. Bathing and the use of cosmetics were undoubtedly part of the category of deeds to be deplored.

However, to counterbalance this, the Crusaders who returned from fighting in odd corners of the Middle East carried with them the cosmetic lore picked up from contact with the local people, mostly feminine. They learned about tooth cleaners, for instance, as well as about using sandstone and pumice to remove unwanted hair.

As the Middle Ages moved on, there were continuing conflicts between the Church's condemnation of the use of cosmetics and the populace's use of them for quite practical reasons. With bathing at an all-time low, the use of perfumed rosewater was an urgent necessity for anyone appearing in public or in small, intimate groups. Still, the sale of cosmetics was thought in many quarters to be the work of the devil enticing man to forget his soul by overconcern for his (or her) body; and those who used them were suspected of witchery. But despite all this disapproval, prostitutes continued to use cosmetics to help their clientele identify them in the public places they frequented. In England rouge was sold in a few shops to trusted customers.

During the frequent plagues that swept Europe, a popular protection was to dip cloth in vinegar, colognes, and perfumes and hold them to the nose and mouth. Perhaps these crude masks did filter out some of the microorganisms causing the Black Death, though no proof is available to show that they did. However, the practice made the smell of unwashed bodies less distressing, and contributed to the ultimate acceptance of cosmetics by conditioning people to accept pleasant and exotic smells.

THE MIDDLE AGES

In the 1500s and 1600s the use of scents of different kinds increased. Clothing was scented—in England most often with lavender, and on the Continent with roses. Rosewater and lavender water were used about the home to remove the unpleasant odors arising from spoiled food, unwashed bodies, and lack of toilet facilities.

At about this time Englishwomen of the more affluent classes began to apply cosmetics habitually. Queen Elizabeth I, a convinced user of cosmetics in generous amounts, established the custom among all classes. Her own preference made hair dyeing popular, and she was instrumental in the introduction of mouth washes and toothpastes.

Italy, which had reintroduced bathing, became the center of the cosmetic world in the sixteenth century, and the voyages of many of the Venetian explorers and traders provided the rare spices and herbs that were beginning to become commercially important in the manufacture of cosmetics. The Dominican monks in Florence set up a perfumery in the early sixteenth century, based on their knowledge of medicinal plants.

In the 1700s, cosmetics began to find wider acceptance among both men and women in Europe. Generally women were more likely to use rouge, skin whiteners made of lead compounds, and perfumes. Perfume shops began to appear, and the ideal of some of the social leaders was not only to find a new perfume, but to use a different one each day of the week. Rouge, to simulate the glow of health in pale and undernourished people, made its debut. Paper leaves sprinkled with carmine were used to brush the cheeks. A favorite form of rouge was "Spanish wool," made of a rough wool, possibly goat, dipped in ocher, a reddish clay. Men used perfumed water on their clothes and on handkerchiefs which they delicately held in front of their noses for obvious reasons. Baths were still not popular, but a well-liked cleanser was almond cream. Soap was more of a curiosity than a household item.

During the 1700s, the fashion focused on women's breasts, and ladies spent much time and effort making the visible areas white; they used rice powder, which frequently caused skin eruptions. Hair oils and pomades were also in vogue, but sometimes made a mess in warm rooms by running and dripping on the wearer.

Actually the French, both men and women, used cosmetics far more than the English—rouge, face and breast powder, oils and pomades for the hair, and flower waters.

Most of us remember the childhood ditty "Yankee Doodle": "Yankee Doodle . . . stuck a feather in his hat and called it Macaroni." Macaroni was not a kind of noodle, but a group of English fops who went around with fantastic hairdos, used cosmetics generously to make their cheeks red, and were not shy about using perfumes. They were in their heyday in the late 1700s and, although they seemed to be aping women in their use of cosmetics, their contemporaries did not consider them deviates.

In a sort of death-rattle attempt to stem the tide of fashion, the British Parliament in 1770 saw the introduction of this infamous (and justly defeated) Bill: "That all women, of whatever rank, profession or

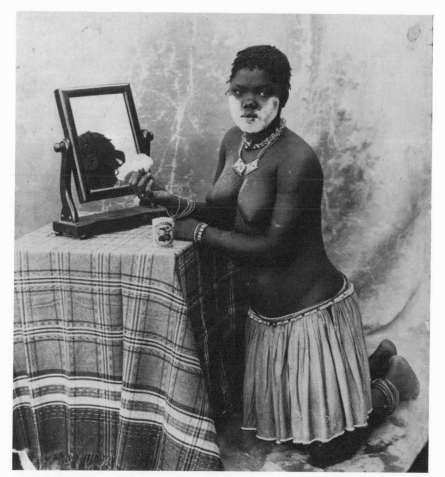

South Africa; Zulu.   Girl kneeling on floor, applying "face powder" in front of a mirror.   Smithsonian Anthropological Archives Negative No. 72-8894 (taken 1890–1910).

degree, whether virgins, maids or widows, that shall from and after such Act, impose upon, seduce and betray into matrimony, any of his Majesty's subjects by the scents, paints, cosmetic washes, artificial teeth, false hair, Spanish wool, iron stays, hoops, high-heeled shoes, and bolstered hips, shall incur the penalty of the law now in force against witchcraft and like misdemeanours, and that the marriage upon conviction shall be null and void."

At the same time there was a gradual popularization of bathing, changes of clothing, and in general a growing concern with the elimination of some of the more noxious body odors and improvement of personal health habits.

TODAY

Today cosmetics have become thoroughly respectable throughout the world, although favored items change from time to time; for example, hair dyes give way, to some extent, to wigs. But there is no decrease in cosmetic use, just a shift in emphasis from time to time.

SHAVING

Since shaving and after-shaving preparations are cosmetics, they also deserve some comment.

Shaving has been a part of man's way of life from prehistoric times. Our primitive ancestors used clam shells, shark's teeth, and sharpened flints to remove whiskers. Egyptian tombs have yielded copper and gold razors from the time of the pharaohs. During the Iron Age, from about 2000 B.C. to around the time of the destruction of Pompeii, warriors were often buried not only with their weapons, but also with their razors. The Romans first considered razors as a symbol of degeneracy.

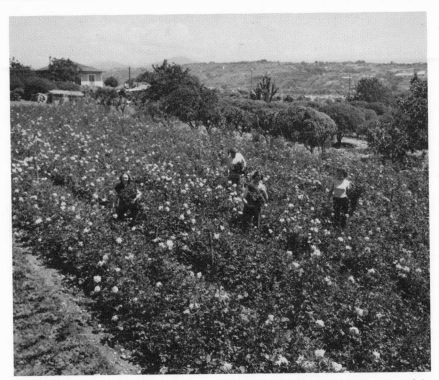

In Provence, near the French Riviera, roses are a major crop, and are used in French perfumery. France Actuelle.

However, as foreigners moved into Rome, many of whom were clean shaven, barber shops soon appeared, and were used by Romans too poor to own slaves to shave them. Alexander the Great, Julius Caesar, and most Roman leaders were clean shaven.

Clean-shaven men have been more frequent in history than bearded men. Perhaps the earliest cave dwellers found a beard too easy to be grabbed by an enemy. Even American Indians were always clean shaven. Traditionally, they plucked out the facial hairs with clam shells.

In Europe in the Middle Ages, barbers were also surgeons, and the red-and-white striped barber pole we know now symbolized the blood and bandages associated with surgery. During this period barbers were permitted to pull teeth and let blood, usually with leeches. Not until the mid-1700s were barbers and surgeons separated profession-ally, to develop their own specialized skills. At this time surgeons were banned from barbering and shaving people.

Our American Revolutionary leaders were clean shaven, as were the British generals. Then the fashion changed, the circle turned, and the Civil War saw mutton chops, beards, and sideburns (named for General Burnside). Photographs of kaisers and czars, kings and em-perors in the 1800s and early 1900s show a variety of beards, mus-taches, and sideburns, but beards were not common during World Wars I and II.

Today men, often younger men, are beginning to grow beards again, but most Americans and Europeans are still clean shaven, with sideburns a little longer than a few years ago.

Beards or not, men still use shaving preparations and after-shave lotions, and will undoubtedly continue to do so.

CONCLUSION

The growing concern with arts and crafts extends to the home produc-tion of personal cosmetics, and creating, shaping, and developing a product to one's own design, using ingredients that are exactly what the maker chooses to use, can be a satisfying hobby. A gift of home-made cosmetics is like any handicraft, a gift of one's own self.

Methods & Materials

Many of the ingredients used in these recipes are available at your local drugstore or supermarket. Others may be obtained from drug distributors or from specialty houses, and I find the "health" stores good sources. Listed in the Appendix are some sources that I have used and found highly satisfactory.

MATERIALS NEEDED

The equipment needed is simple. The basic tools are measuring cups; measuring spoons; a simple strainer or a hand-operated colander; pieces of cheesecloth, muslin, and nylon; a couple of pots in which to warm materials; a funnel and some filter paper; and a wooden spoon for stirring ingredients. A blender may be useful at times; a grinder may help; and bottles and jars for storing materials would complete the list. I have done my work in the basement of our home on a simple table made of an old wooden door, with four folding legs. A hot plate is helpful if you work away from the kitchen area.

Distilled water is preferred wherever water is listed in recipes, though it is not an absolute necessity. Distilled water is often available at drugstores; at garages (where it is called battery water); and in bottles at many supermarkets.

ALCOHOL

I have used two kinds of alcohols. Isopropyl, the familiar rubbing alcohol (70 percent alcohol) is usable for all external applications, but not for mouth washes and other preparations taken orally. Ethyl alcohol can be substituted for isopropyl if one desires. However, isopropyl must never be substituted for ethyl alcohol for mouth washes and internal use.

Ethyl alcohol can be bought at strengths up to 100 percent, which are extremely expensive. For use in cosmetics, 95 percent ethyl alcohol is suitable (see the table on page 220 for help in converting to lower strengths). In the recipes where no type of alcohol is specified, isopropyl or ethyl alcohols can be used usually at 70 percent. How-

13

ever, with experience the percentages can be changed to meet individual tastes.

Isopropyl alcohol is a petroleum by-product; ethyl alcohol can be made from fruits and grains, although most of it is made from blackstrap molasses. Some may be made from sawdust, some from petroleum.

In heating alcohol or alcohol-based materials, like witch hazel, always use a water bath for safety. Put the alcohol in a small pot and then place the small pot in the larger pot of water.

While aging or steeping materials, be sure they are covered, to reduce loss by evaporation and to keep dust out.

PROCEDURES

Be thorough in mixing, blending, and combining ingredients. All the oils listed are first combined with alcohol because this enables them to go into solution and makes mixing easier. Usually one teaspoon of oil is dissolved in a cup of alcohol.

I have used "kitchen" measurements rather than the more formal grams, milliliters, and such to facilitate compounding and to eliminate the cost of special scales, balances, and measuring devices.

The recipes I have listed are flexible, and the amounts used can be varied as the user becomes familiar with the results of the work.

Solids, such as soaps and cocoa butter, can be measured simply by displacement. For example, if 1/4 cup of cocoa butter is required, fill a measuring cup with water to the 3/4 cup mark and add cocoa butter until the water measures 1 cup. If 1 1/2 cups are required, a larger measuring bowl can be used in the same way; or 3 1/2 cups of the solid can be measured one at a time.

SUBSTITUTIONS

Even the ingredients can be varied to meet availability and personal preference. For example, when I have needed a mucilage, I have used Irish moss tea instead of Irish moss (simply because Irish moss tea is sold in a local health store) with excellent results. Denture adhesive powders have gums, like karaya, which can be used in cosmetic work.

STRAINER OR FILTER?

Whether to strain with a strainer or a cheesecloth or to use a filter will depend on the size of the particles to be removed. Finer, more liquid solutions can go through filter paper readily. Thicker solutions,

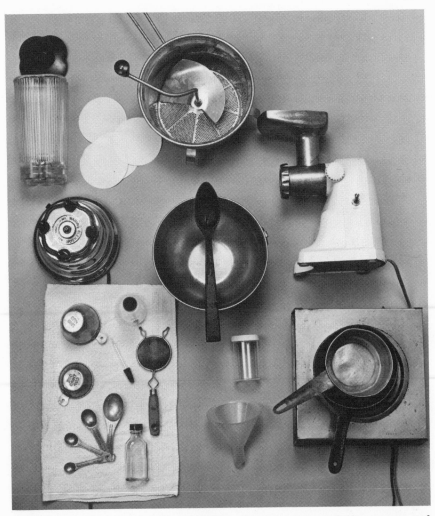

These are the tools I use in my cosmetic work. Only the round filter papers and plastic vials are somewhat unusual among kitchen utensils. Medicine bottles can be washed and saved. A water bath is made by setting one pot in another. W. Uzzle.

with larger pieces, will hardly go through a filter but can go through a strainer or cheesecloth.

NAMES

I have found that some confusion exists in the use of certain terms. Such words as *essence*, *extract*, *spirit*, and others mean exactly the same thing—an alcoholic solution of the volatile oils used in perfumery. An *extract* is any material which has been extracted from plant materials by one of a variety of methods. Extract of witch hazel and extract of vanilla are two familiar examples. The plant material is steeped in a suitable liquid. If the liquid is alcohol the resulting extract may be called *essence*, *spirit*, *otto*, or *attar*. These are usually essential oils (volatile oils).

Indeed, it is nice to know that volatile oil and essential oil mean the same thing—the aromatic oil of a plant, usually extracted by distillation but sometimes by other methods. *Enfleurage*, for example, used in France, is the mixing of rose petals with the best quality of oil to extract the essential oil.

A *tincture* is made by steeping a part of a plant, like the vanilla bean, in alcohol to extract the desired scents.

Because these are natural cosmetics without emulsifiers, thickeners, and such additions, the finished product may not resemble some of the commercial products you are familiar with in stores. Just remember that, regardless of appearance, the purpose for which you made the cosmetics is being met.

Astringent Lotions, Skin Fresheners, Friction Lotions

Skin fresheners, friction lotions, and astringent lotions have similar uses. Applied to the skin, they add moisture and aid in keeping the skin smooth.

An *astringent lotion* causes the pores to shrink or contract, and helps to minimize blackheads and skin blemishes. It is useful in treating oily skin. It may contain a combination of a number of ingredients with astringent qualities, including alcohol, witch hazel, alum, lemon juice, and vinegar.

A *skin freshener* contains up to 15 percent alcohol, while a *friction lotion* may contain as much as 50 percent. As they are rubbed into the skin the alcohol evaporates, leaving the moisture for the skin to absorb. The skin is left smooth and fresh smelling. Both friction lotions and skin fresheners may contain astringents, most commonly witch hazel.

These preparations have a long history. Aromatic water, usually rosewater, was applied to the skin after bathing by the Greeks, Romans, and the East Indians. All were widely used during the Middle Ages, before bathing became popular and fashionable in Europe.

CAMPHOR WATER ASTRINGENT LOTION

Camphor	1/8 teaspoon
Alcohol	1 teaspoon
Water	1 cup

☞ Dissolve the camphor in the alcohol. Add the water.

17

CUCUMBER ASTRINGENT LOTION

Cucumber juice	1/4 cup plus 2 tablespoons
Cologne water	1/4 cup (see Ch. 6, Colognes)
Tincture of benzoin	2 tablespoons
Elder-flower water	1 cup

☞ Slice 1/2 large, unpeeled cucumber into 1/4 cup warm water. Let set until the cucumber becomes pulpy. Squeeze the mixture through muslin to remove the juice. Discard the pulp. Combine the juice with the other ingredients.

LEMON ASTRINGENT LOTION

Alum	1 teaspoon
Boric acid powder	1/2 teaspoon
Fresh lemon juice	1/4 cup
Witch hazel	1/2 cup
Alcohol	1/2 cup

☞ Combine the ingredients.

ORANGE-FLOWER ASTRINGENT LOTION

Alum	1/4 teaspoon
Cologne water	1/4 cup plus 2 teaspoons
Orange-flower water	1 1/2 cups plus 2 tablespoons

☞ Dissolve the alum in the cologne water. Add the orange-flower water.

ROSEWATER ASTRINGENT LOTION

Alum	4 tablespoons
Potassium carbonate	1 tablespoon
Glycerin	1 tablespoon
Rosewater	1 1/4 cups

☞ Mix the alum and the potassium carbonate with the rosewater. Add the glycerin.

STRAWBERRY ASTRINGENT LOTION

Strawberries, mashed	1/2 cup
White wine vinegar	1/2 cup
Rosewater	1/2 cup

☛ Mix the strawberries and vinegar in a bottle and let set overnight. Strain to remove the strawberry pulp, and add the rosewater.

VIOLET WITCH HAZEL ASTRINGENT LOTION

Tincture of rose geranium	2 tablespoons
Witch hazel	1 cup
Oil of jasmine	1/4 teaspoon
Oil of orris	1/8 teaspoon
Alcohol	1 tablespoon

☛ Dissolve the oils in the alcohol. Add the remaining ingredients.

WITCH HAZEL ASTRINGENT LOTION

Alcohol	2 tablespoons
Witch hazel	1 cup

☛ Combine the ingredients.

ALMOND-ROSE SKIN FRESHENER

Borax	1 teaspoon
Tincture of benzoin	1 1/2 teaspoons
Rosewater	1 cup
Almonds, sliced	2 teaspoons
Water	1/4 cup

☛ Dissolve the borax in the tincture of benzoin. Add the rosewater. Combine the almonds and water in a blender, and add to the rosewater mixture.

ORANGE BLOSSOM SKIN FRESHENER

Borax	1 teaspoon
Tincture of benzoin	1 teaspoon
Water	3/4 cup
Oil of neroli	1/4 teaspoon

☞ Dissolve the borax and the oil in the tincture. Add the water.

ROSE SKIN FRESHENER

Borax	1 teaspoon
Camphor	1/4 teaspoon
Tincture of benzoin	1 1/2 teaspoons
Rosewater	1/2 cup
Water	1 cup

☞ Dissolve the borax and camphor in the tincture. Add the rosewater and the water.

WITCH HAZEL SKIN FRESHENER

Alcohol	3/4 cup
Glycerin	2 teaspoons
Oil of jasmine	5 drops
Witch hazel	2 teaspoons

☞ Combine all the ingredients, and shake well to mix.

ORANGE-FLOWER WATER FRICTION LOTION

Boric acid powder	1/2 teaspoon
Witch hazel	1 tablespoon
Rosewater	1 tablespoon
Alcohol	2 teaspoons
Orange-flower water	1/4 cup

☞ Dissolve the boric acid in the alcohol. Add the other ingredients. Let set for a week before using.

ROSE SKIN-TONING LOTION

Boric acid powder	1/4 teaspoon
Witch hazel	1 tablespoon
Rosewater	1/4 cup
Alcohol	2 teaspoons

☛ Dissolve the boric acid in the alcohol. Add the other ingredients. Let set for a week before using.

Bath Preparations

Bath preparations are of several types. There are bath oils, milks, ammonia waters and vinegars, salts, bubble baths, bath oatmeals, and various herbal bath bags.

There are two major kinds of bath oils. One is soluble in water, while the other floats on the surface of the water, leaving its drops evenly distributed on the skin.

Ammonia water, bubble bath, and salts all have a dual purpose, softening the water and cleansing the skin at the same time.

The various bath bags, made up of different grains and dried herbs, and the bath oatmeal are very gentle to the skin as well as cleansing.

Bran water, oatmeal water, and other grains are good for sensitive skins. The various ammonia waters and toilet vinegars are both cleansing and deodorizing. Many of the herbs and barks included here contain saponins, which have the effect of soap.

Some of these bath preparations have been held in esteem for thousands of years. Poppaea, the wife of Nero, bathed in asses' milk, as did Cleopatra and Isabeau, wife of King Charles VI of France. Mary, Queen of Scots, bathed in wine. Since soap was not widely used in Europe until the seventeenth century, it is possible that all these bath preparations were meant to be cleansers.

BATH PREPARATIONS

BALSAM BATH OIL

Oil of nutmeg	2 teaspoons
Oil of pine	3 tablespoons
Oil of cloves	2 tablespoons
Oil of cassie	2 tablespoons
Peru balsam	1/4 cup
Tincture of benzoin	1/4 cup

☞ Combine the ingredients.

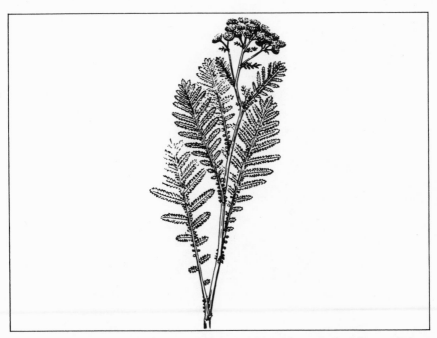

Tansy is a perennial, two to three feet in height, with aromatic foliage. It is a weed found in dry areas in many parts of the United States. It is used in sachets, bath preparations, and facial packs. (Tanacetum vulgare) University of West Virginia.

CLOVE BATH OIL

Oil of lemon	1 tablespoon
Oil of sandalwood	1 tablespoon
Oil of cedarwood	1 tablespoon
Oil of cloves	1 1/2 tablespoons
Castor oil	1 cup

☞ Combine the ingredients.

EUCALYPTUS BATH OIL

Eucalyptol	1/3 cup plus 1 teaspoon
Castor oil	1 1/2 cup plus 1 tablespoon

☞ Combine the ingredients.

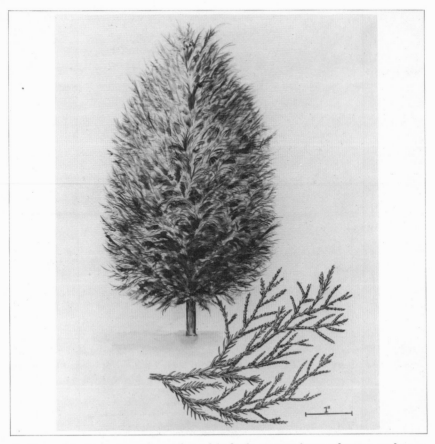

Cedarwood is the source of an oil used in bath preparations, colognes, and soap. Cedarwood chips are used in sachets. (Juniperus virginiana) U.S. Forest Service.

PINE BATH OIL [1]

Olive oil	1 1/2 cups
Alcohol	4 tablespoons
Oil of pine	2 tablespoons

☞ Mix the olive oil and the oil of pine. Add the alcohol.

PINE BATH OIL [2]

Oil of pine	1 tablespoon
Castor oil	1/4 cup
Pine-needle resin	1/4 cup

| Alcohol | 2 tablespoons |
| Olive oil | 1 1/4 cups |

☞ Dissolve the oil of pine and the resin in the alcohol.   Add the castor oil and olive oil.

PINE-EUCALYPTUS BATH MILK

Tincture of benzoin	1 1/2 tablespoons
Alcohol	1 1/2 cups
Water	1 1/2 cups
Oil of eucalyptus	10 drops
Oil of lemon	1/8 teaspoon
Oil of pine	1/4 teaspoon

☞ Dissolve the oils in the alcohol.   Combine with the tincture and water.   Use 1/2 cup per bath.

PINE BATH MILK

Soap flakes	1 tablespoon
Alcohol	3/4 cup
Tragacanth	2 tablespoons
Oil of pine	3 tablespoons
Water, hot	4 1/2 cups

☞ Dissolve the soap in the water.   Add the tragacanth and mix to a smooth paste.   Dissolve the oil in the alcohol and add to the water mixture.   Use about 1/4 cup for each bath, adding directly under the running water.

MILK BATH

Powdered milk	1/3 cup
Gelatin	2 tablespoons
Epsom salts	1 cup
Powdered hops	1/4 cup
Elder flowers	1/4 cup

☞ Combine the ingredients.   Use 1/2 cup per bath.

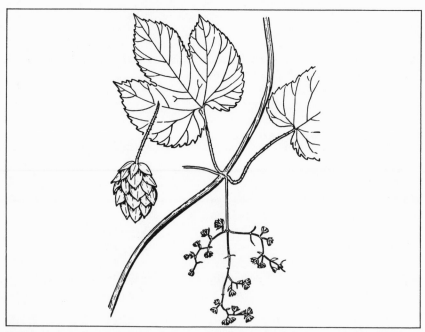

Hops are most famous for the part they play in beer-making. The twining peren-nials are cultivated and also grow wild in the eastern two-thirds of the United States. An oil from the plant is used in colognes and perfumes. The dried hop, a flower which has a conelike shape, is used in herbal bath preparations and facial masks. (Humulus spp.) University of West Virginia.

OATMEAL BATH BAGS

Oatmeal	3 1/2 cups
Bran	1 cup
Orrisroot powder	4 tablespoons
Soap flakes	3 tablespoons
Orange sachet powder	1 1/2 teaspoons

☛ Grind the oatmeal and the bran in a blender until fine. Add to the other ingredients. Tie up in cheesecloth bags in 1/4 cup portions. Then tie the bag on the faucet and let it hang down so the running water will flow through it.

HERBAL BATH BAGS

Rosemary	1 cup
Dill herb	1 cup

| Mint, dried | 1 cup |
| Linden flowers, dried | 1 cup |

☞ Combine the ingredients. Tie in cheesecloth bags, 1/2 cup to a bag. Use in the same way as oatmeal bath bags.

BRAN BATH BAGS

Orrisroot powder	1/2 cup
Bran	1 cup
Myrrh, powdered	1/4 cup
Powdered milk	1/2 cup
Alum	1/4 teaspoon

☞ Combine and tie up in cheesecloth bags in portions of 1/4 cup. Use like oatmeal bath bags.

VIOLET BATH BAGS

Oatmeal, finely ground	3 cups
Orrisroot powder	1/4 cup plus 2 tablespoons
Almond meal	1/4 cup
Soap flakes	1/2 cup

☞ Tie up in cheesecloth bags. Use as directed under other bath bags.

THE PERFUMED BATH FOR WOMEN IN MERRIE ENGLAND

"A SWEET-SCENTED BATH"

☞ "Roses, Citron flowers, Orange flowers, Jasmine, Bays, Rosemary, Lavender, Mint, Pennyroyal, and Citron peel, each a sufficient quantity, boyl them together gently, and make a bath, to which add Oyl of Spike 6 drops, Musk 5 grains, Ambergrease 3 grains, sweet Asa 1 ounce. Let her go into the Bath before meat." [Ca. 1400]

HERBAL BATH

☞ "Take rosemary, Feverfew, Orgaine, Pellitory of the wall, Fennell, Mallowes, Violet leaves and nettles, boil all these together, and when it is well sodden, put to it two or three gallons of milk, then let the party stand or sit in it for an hour or two, the bath reaching up to the stomach and when they come out they must go to bed and sweat, and beware taking of cold." [Ca. 1500]

Any of the following may be used in bath bags. All must be thoroughly dried and cured before they are suitable for use.

Barley   *Hordeum* spp.
Burnet   *Sanguisorba officinalis*
Comfrey root   *Symphytum officinale*
Dill   *Anethum graveolens*
Elder flowers   *Sambucus canadensis*
Eucalyptus   *Eucalyptus globulus*
Fennel   *Foeniculum vulgare*
Hops   *Humulus lupulus*
Horsetails   *Equisetum arvense*
Laurel   *Laurus nobilis*
Lemon balm   *Melissa officinalis*
Linden flowers   *Lindera benzoin*
Lovage   *Levisticum officinale*
Peppermint   *Mentha piperita*
Rosebuds and petals   *Rosa* spp.
Rosemary   *Rosmarinus officinalis*
Sage   *Salvia officinalis*
Thyme   *Thymus vulgaris*
Woodruff   *Asperula odorata*
Yarrow   *Achillea millefolium*

BATH SALTS [1]

Soap flakes	3/4 cup
Borax	1/2 cup
Extract of jasmine	1 1/2 tablespoons

☞ Combine the soap and borax. Add the jasmine extract, and stir until the alcohol evaporates. Use a heaping tablespoon per bath.

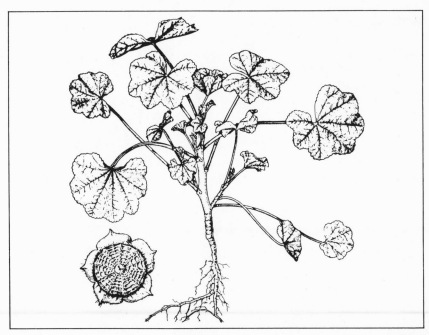

Mallows are found wild and cultivated, growing from one to eight feet in height. They are very mucilaginous and emollient, and are used in lotions, facial masks, creams, and herbal baths. (Malva spp.) University of Arizona.

BATH SALTS [2]

Borax	3/4 cup
Extract of cassie	1 teaspoon
Extract of jasmine	1 teaspoon
Oil of lavender	1/8 teaspoon

☛ Rub the oil and the extracts with the borax until the alcohol evaporates. Use a heaping tablespoon per bath.

BATH SALTS [3]

Borax	1/3 cup
Potassium carbonate	1/2 cup
Almond meal	1/2 cup
Oil of cinnamon	1 teaspoon
Oil of eucalyptus	1 teaspoon

☛ Combine the dry ingredients. Stir in the oils. Use a heaping tablespoon per bath.

BATH SALTS [4]

Soap flakes	1/2 cup
Sodium carbonate	2 teaspoons
Orrisroot powder	3 tablespoons
Almond meal	3 tablespoons
Oil of bergamot	5 drops
Oil of lemon	1/8 teaspoon
Oil of cloves	7 drops

☞ Combine the dry ingredients. Add the oils. Use a heaping tablespoon per bath.

LAVENDER-AMMONIA BATH WATER

Ammonia water	1 cup
Water	3/4 cup plus 2 tablespoons
Alcohol	2 tablespoons
Oil of lavender	1/4 teaspoon

☞ Dissolve the oil in the alcohol. Mix with the water and the ammonia water. Use 1/2 cup per bath.

AMMONIA BATH WATER WITH SOAP

Ammonia water	1 cup
Soap flakes	1/2 cup
Water, hot	1 cup
Borax	1/2 cup
Potassium carbonate	1/2 cup

☞ Dissolve the soap, borax, and potassium carbonate in the water. Add the ammonia water. Use 1/2 cup per bath.

AMMONIA BATH WATER WITH COLOGNE

Ammonia water	1 1/2 cups
Soap flakes	3/4 cup
Borax	1 1/2 tablespoons
Cologne water	3 tablespoons
Water, hot	1 1/4 cups

☞ Dissolve the soap and borax in the water. Add the cologne water, then the ammonia water. Use 1/2 cup per bath.

BORÀTED BATHING SOLUTION

Boric acid powder	1 tablespoon
Alum	1 1/2 teaspoons
Camphor	1 1/2 teaspoons
Alcohol	1/2 cup
Water	2 cups

☛ Dissolve the boric acid, alum, and camphor in the alcohol and add the water. Use 1 cup per bath.

VIOLET-AMMONIA BATH WATER [1]

Ammonia water	2/3 cup
Water	2/3 cup
Tincture of orris	2 tablespoons

☛ Combine the water and the tincture. Add the ammonia water. Use 1/2 cup per bath.

VIOLET-AMMONIA BATH WATER [2]

Ammonia water	3/4 cup plus 2 tablespoons
Tincture of orris	2 tablespoons
Alcohol	2 tablespoons
Water	3 cups

☛ Combine the tincture, alcohol, and water. Add the ammonia water. Use 3/4 cup per bath.

SCENTED BUBBLE BATH

Soap flakes	1 1/2 cups
Water, hot	2 cups
Glycerin	1/4 cup
Alcohol	2 tablespoons
Oil of sandalwood	1/4 teaspoon
Oil of strawberry	1/2 teaspoon

☛ Dissolve the oils in the alcohol and add the glycerin. Dissolve the soap in the water and combine with the alcohol mixture. Store in a wide-mouthed jar for convenience. Use about 2 tablespoons for each bath.

AFTER-BATH DUSTING POWDERS

The purpose of dusting powder is to absorb moisture and to keep the skin smelling fresh and feeling smooth. It can be scented, unscented, or medicated, and may be made of a variety of materials, including talc, chalk, fine flours, starch, fuller's earth, and mixtures of these.

ANTISEPTIC DUSTING POWDER

Talc	2 tablespoons
Boric acid powder	1 tablespoon
Rice flour	1/2 cup

☞ Combine the ingredients.

BLUEBERRY TALC

Talc	2 cups
Magnesium carbonate	3 tablespoons
Boric acid powder	2 tablespoons
Oil of blueberry	1 teaspoon

☞ Combine the powders; add the oil.

CASSIE DUSTING POWDER

Rice flour	1/4 cup
Talc	1/4 cup
Orrisroot powder	2 tablespoons
Cornstarch	1 cup
Extract of jasmine	1 teaspoon
Extract of cassie	1 1/2 teaspoons

☞ Combine the ingredients.

HONEYSUCKLE DUSTING POWDER

Rice flour	1 cup
Cornstarch	1 1/4 cups

| Magnesium carbonate | 1/4 cup |
| Honeysuckle cologne | 2 tablespoons |

☞ Combine the dry ingredients and stir in the cologne.

JASMINE DUSTING POWDER

Precipitated chalk	1 cup
Talc	1/4 cup
Orrisroot powder	1 1/2 teaspoons
Boric acid powder	1 1/2 teaspoons
Extract of cassie	1/4 teaspoon
Extract of jasmine	1 teaspoon

☞ Combine the chalk, talc, orrisroot, and boric acid. Stir in the extracts.

LAVENDER TALC

Talc	1 cup
Oil of lavender	10 drops
Oil of rose	5 drops
Oil of cinnamon	1/8 teaspoon

☞ Stir the oils into the talc.

LAVENDER DUSTING POWDER

Talc	1 cup
Cornstarch	1 cup
Oil of lavender	1/8 teaspoon
Oil of rose	10 drops
Oil of cinnamon	1/8 teaspoon

☞ Combine the talc and cornstarch. Stir in the oils.

COOLING MENTHOLATED TALC

Menthol	1/2 teaspoon
Alcohol	1 teaspoon
Talc	1 cup

☞ Dissolve the menthol in the alcohol. Mix with the talc.

NEROLI TALC

Talc	1 3/4 cups
Boric acid powder	1/3 cup
Oil of neroli	1 teaspoon

☞ Combine the talc and boric acid. Stir in the oil.

NEROLI DUSTING POWDER

Talc	1/2 cup
Kaolin	1 cup
Boric acid powder	1 tablespoon
Oil of sandalwood	1/8 teaspoon
Oil of clove	10 drops

☞ Combine the talc, kaolin, and boric acid powder. Stir in the oils.

TEA ROSE TALC

Talc	2 cups
Oil of rose	5 drops
Oil of wintergreen	1 drop
Extract of jasmine	1 teaspoon

☞ Dissolve the oils in the jasmine extract, and add to the talc.

ROSE DUSTING POWDER

Talc	1 cup
Cornstarch	1 cup
Oil of rose	1/2 teaspoon

☞ Combine the talc and cornstarch. Stir in the oil.

ROSE GERANIUM DUSTING POWDER

Boric acid powder	3 tablespoons
Starch	1/4 cup

| Talc | 1 cup |
| Oil of rose geranium | 1/2 teaspoon |

☞ Combine the boric acid, starch, and talc. Add the oil.

STRAWBERRY BATH POWDER

Talc	2 cups
Boric acid powder	3 tablespoons
Starch	1/4 cup
Oil of strawberry	1 teaspoon

☞ Combine the powders, and add the oil.

BERGAMOT-VIOLET DUSTING POWDER

Orrisroot powder	1 tablespoon
Cornstarch	1 cup
Oil of bergamot	10 drops
Oil of orange	3 drops

☞ Combine the orrisroot and cornstarch. Stir in the oils.

CITRUS-VIOLET DUSTING POWDER

Starch	1 cup
Talc	1 tablespoon
Orrisroot powder	1/2 tablespoon
Oil of bergamot	10 drops
Oil of lemon grass	10 drops
Oil of bitter almond	3 drops

☞ Combine the starch, orrisroot, and talc. Stir in the oils.

JASMINE-VIOLET TALC

Talc	1/2 cup
Orrisroot powder	3 tablespoons
Extract of jasmine	1/4 teaspoon

☞ Combine the talc and orrisroot. Stir in the extract.

LEMON-VIOLET BATH POWDER

Cornstarch	2 cups
Orrisroot powder	1 tablespoon
Oil of lemon	1/4 teaspoon
Oil of neroli	10 drops
Oil of jasmine	5 drops

☞ Combine the cornstarch and orrisroot. Add the oils and stir.

VIOLET TALC

Talc	2 1/4 cups
Boric acid powder	1/4 cup
Orrisroot powder	2 tablespoons
Extract of orris	1 1/2 tablespoons

☞ Combine the powders and stir in the extract.

VIOLET DUSTING POWDER

Talc	1/2 cup
Starch	1 cup
Orrisroot powder	1/2 cup
Oil of orris	10 drops

☞ Combine the powders, then stir in the oil.

UNSCENTED BATH POWDER [1]

Rice flour	3/4 cup
Cornstarch	3 cups

☞ Combine the ingredients.

UNSCENTED BATH POWDER [2]

Talc	2 cups
Boric acid powder	2 teaspoons
Magnesium carbonate	1 tablespoon

☞ Combine the ingredients.

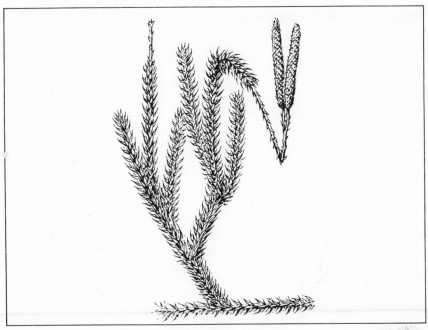

Lycopodium, or club moss, is a small, mosslike plant that grows almost flat on the ground all over the United States. The spores are powdery and are used in dusting powders. (Lycopodium spp.) University of West Virginia.

ROSE BABY POWDER

Talc	2 cups
Fuller's earth	1/2 cup
Lycopodium powder	1/2 cup
Oil of rose	10 drops

☛ Combine the talc, fuller's earth, and lycopodium powder. Stir in the oil.

BABY POWDER WITH OLIVE OIL

Fuller's earth	1 1/4 cups
Talc	3/4 cup
Cornstarch	3/4 cup
Olive oil	2 tablespoons

☛ Combine the fuller's earth, talc, and cornstarch. Mix in the olive oil.

UNSCENTED BABY POWDER

Fuller's earth	1 1/4 cup
Cornstarch	2 cups
Talc	3/4 cup

☞ Combine the ingredients.

Cold Creams & Cleansing Creams

Cleansing cream is used to remove makeup, surface dirt, and oil from the face and throat. The cream does this by forming an emulsion with the oil and dirt on the face. It is also a source of moisture for the skin.

The first cold cream was made by the Greek physician Galen around 150 A.D. It consisted of an emulsion of beeswax, olive oil, animal fat, and vegetable oils. Unlike modern cold creams, it turned rancid, separated, and took a lot of time to manufacture.

Because women could use cold cream without social criticism, moisturizing creams formed the basis for one of the first cosmetic companies operating on a commercial level, that of the famous Helena Rubinstein.

Some of the cleansing creams I have included take more preparation than others, because the different waxes and fats must be melted and mixed carefully at specified temperatures in order to form an emulsion. Other creams and jellies are fairly simple in ingredients and procedure, and are marvelous for special skin problems because they are so gentle.

CLEANSING LOTIONS

BENZOIN CLEANSING MILK

Tincture of benzoin	2 tablespoons
Alcohol	1/4 cup
Glycerin	1/4 cup
Water	1 1/2 cups

☛ Combine ingredients.

COCOA BUTTER CLEANSING MILK [1]

Borax	1/2 teaspoon
Cocoa butter	1 teaspoon
Coconut oil	1 teaspoon
Rosewater	1 cup
Liquid soap	1 teaspoon

☞ Melt the cocoa butter and coconut oil together. Add the borax, and stir until it dissolves. Stir in the rosewater gradually and then add the soap.

COCOA BUTTER CLEANSING MILK [2]

Borax	1/2 teaspoon
Soap flakes	1 1/2 tablespoons
Coconut oil	2 teaspoons
Water	3/4 cup
Cocoa butter	1/4 cup
Rosewater	1 cup
Oil of bitter almond	5 drops
Oil of bergamot	1/8 teaspoon

☞ Dissolve the cocoa butter, coconut oil, and borax over low heat. Add the soap. Warm the water and rosewater to lukewarm and add to the first mixture. Stir in the scented oils.

CUCUMBER CLEANSING MILK [1]

Almond oil	1 tablespoon
Soap flakes	1 teaspoon
Tincture of benzoin	1/2 teaspoon
Cucumbers	2
Water, hot	1 1/2 cups

☞ Pour the water over the sliced, unpeeled cucumbers. When they become pulpy, squeeze through muslin to remove the juice. Combine the juice, almond oil, soap, and tincture.

CUCUMBER CLEANSING MILK [2]

Cucumber	1
Water, hot	3/4 cup
Almond oil	1/4 cup
Liquid soap	1 tablespoon
Tincture of benzoin	1 teaspoon
Oil of bitter almond	5 drops
Oil of lavender	1/8 teaspoon

☛ Make the cucumber juice as directed in the previous formula. Dissolve the scents in the tincture, and add the remaining ingredients.

CUCUMBER CLEANSING MILK [3]

Almonds, sliced	1/4 cup
Cucumber	1
Water, hot	1 cup
Liquid soap	1 tablespoon
Tincture of benzoin	1 teaspoon
Rosewater	1/4 cup

☛ Make the cucumber juice as directed under Cucumber Cleansing Milk [1]. Place the almonds in a blender with the rosewater, and blend to make a milk. Combine this with the cucumber juice. Add the soap and tincture of benzoin.

GLYCERIN-LANOLIN CLEANSING MILK

Lanolin	1/4 cup
Glycerin	1/4 cup
Tincture of benzoin	3 tablespoons
Irish moss	2 teaspoons
Water	2 cups

☛ Boil the Irish moss with the water to form a mucilage. Melt the lanolin over low heat, and add the glycerin. Combine with the mucilage, and stir in the tincture of benzoin.

LANOLIN CLEANSING MILK [1]

Lanolin	2 tablespoons
Soap flakes	2 tablespoons
Tincture of benzoin	1 teaspoon
Water, hot	2 cups

☞ Melt the lanolin over low heat. Dissolve the soap in the water and add to the lanolin. Stir in the tincture of benzoin.

LANOLIN CLEANSING MILK [2]

Lanolin	2 teaspoons
Soap flakes	1 teaspoon
Glycerin	2 teaspoons
Rosewater	1/2 cup
Tincture of benzoin	1/2 teaspoon
Water, hot	1 cup

☞ Melt the lanolin over low heat. Dissolve the soap in the water and add to the lanolin. Stir in the remaining ingredients.

ROSE LANOLIN CLEANSING MILK

Lanolin	2 tablespoons
Soap flakes	1/2 teaspoon
Glycerin	1 tablespoon
Rosewater	3/4 cup
Tincture of benzoin	1 teaspoon
Water, hot	1 1/4 cups

☞ Melt the lanolin over low heat. Dissolve the soap in the water and add the lanolin. Stir in the remaining ingredients.

ROSE CLEANSING MILK [1]

Tincture of benzoin	1 tablespoon
Tincture of storax	1 1/2 teaspoons
Rosewater	1 cup
Water	1 cup
Alcohol	1/4 cup
Oil of rose	8 drops

☞ Dissolve the oil in the alcohol. Add the remaining ingredients.

ROSE CLEANSING MILK [2]

Almond oil	2 tablespoons
Soap flakes	3 tablespoons
Potassium carbonate	3 tablespoons
Water, hot	1 1/2 cups
Alcohol	1/4 cup
Oil of rose	8 drops
Rosewater	1 cup

☞ Dissolve the soap and potassium carbonate in the water. Add the almond oil. Dissolve the oil of rose in the alcohol, and add to the cooled first mixture. Stir in the rosewater.

CUCUMBER CLEANSING LOTION

Cucumber	1
Water, hot	3/4 cup
Liquid soap	3 tablespoons
Tincture of benzoin	1 teaspoon
Alcohol	1 tablespoon
Oil of lavender	10 drops
Oil of bergamot	1/8 teaspoon

☞ Make the cucumber juice as directed under Cucumber Cleansing Milk [1]. Dissolve the scents in the alcohol. Combine the cucumber juice and the alcohol, and stir in the remaining ingredients.

ORANGE-FLOWER CLEANSING LOTION

Potassium carbonate	1/4 cup
Water	1 cup
Orange-flower water	1/2 cup
Alcohol	1 tablespoon
Tincture of vanilla	1 teaspoon
Oil of neroli	10 drops

☞ Dissolve the potassium carbonate in the water. Add the orange-flower water and the tincture of vanilla. Dissolve the oil of neroli in the alcohol, and add to the first mixture.

QUINCE SEED CLEANSING LOTION

Quince seed	1 1/2 teaspoons
Water, hot	1 cup
Glycerin	1/4 cup
Alcohol	1/4 cup
Oil of rose	10 drops

☞ Combine the quince seed and water and let set to form a mucilage. Strain, then add the glycerin. Dissolve the oil in the alcohol, and add to the first mixture.

CLEANSING JELLIES

AGAR-AGAR JELLY

Agar-agar	1 teaspoon
Glycerin	1/4 cup
Water	3/4 cup

☞ Soak the agar-agar in the water until softened. Bring to a boil over low heat, and stir until the solution becomes clear. Add the glycerin.

AGAR-GELATIN JELLY

Gelatin	1/4 teaspoon
Agar-agar	1/2 teaspoon
Glycerin	2 tablespoons
Water	1/2 cup
Boric acid powder	1/2 teaspoon

☞ Soak the gelatin and agar-agar in the water until softened. Dissolve over low heat, and stir in the glycerin and the boric acid.

ALMOND GLYCERIN JELLY [1]

Soap flakes	1 teaspoon
Water, hot	1 1/2 tablespoons
Glycerin	2 tablespoons
Almond oil	1 cup
Oil of thyme	10 drops

☛ Combine the soap and water. Stir in the glycerin, almond oil, and oil of thyme.

ALMOND GLYCERIN JELLY [2]

Glycerin	1/3 cup
Almond oil	1 cup
Soap flakes	1 teaspoon
Water, hot	1 1/2 tablespoons
Oil of orange	10 drops

☛ Combine the soap, glycerin, and water. Add the almond oil gradually. Stir in the oil of orange.

GLYCERIN CLEANSING JELLY WITH BENZOIN

Tincture of benzoin	2 tablespoons
Glycerin	1/4 cup

☛ Combine ingredients.

ARROWROOT GLYCERIN JELLY

Arrowroot powder	1/2 teaspoon
Water	1/2 cup
Glycerin	1 cup
Boric acid powder	1/2 teaspoon

☛ Combine the arrowroot with the water to form a smooth paste. Stir in the glycerin. Heat, stirring constantly, over low heat until a smooth jelly is formed. Add the boric acid, and stir until it dissolves.

GLYCERIN-STARCH JELLY [1]

Rice flour	1 tablespoon
Glycerin	1/4 cup
Water	2 tablespoons

☞ Mix the flour with the water to form a smooth paste. Add the glycerin, then heat over a water bath until the mixture becomes smooth and clear.

GLYCERIN-STARCH JELLY [2]

Rice flour	2 tablespoons
Glycerin	1/4 cup
Water	1/2 cup

☞ Mix the flour with one tablespoon of the water to form a smooth paste. Add the remaining water and glycerin. Heat, stirring, until smooth and clear.

ALMOND-HONEY JELLY

Honey	1 tablespoon
Glycerin	1 tablespoon
Olive oil	1/2 cup
Almond oil	1/2 cup
Oil of rose	10 drops
Water	1 tablespoon

☞ Combine the honey and glycerin, and stir in the oils. Add the water.

LAVENDER CLEANSING JELLY

Gelatin	2 teaspoons
Glycerin	3/4 cup
Water	1/2 cup
Oil of rose	1 drop
Oil of lavender	1/8 teaspoon

☞ Soak the gelatin in the water to soften. Dissolve over low heat, and stir in the glycerin and oils.

HONEY-GLYCERIN JELLY

Gelatin	1 teaspoon
Honey	2 teaspoons
Glycerin	1/4 cup
Alcohol	1/2 teaspoon
Water	2 tablespoons

☞ Soak the gelatin in the water to soften it. Dissolve over low heat. Cool to lukewarm, and add the remaining ingredients.

LAVENDER-GLYCERIN JELLY

Glycerin	1/2 cup
Honey	1 tablespoon
Water	1 cup
Gelatin	2 teaspoons
Oil of lavender	1/8 teaspoon

☞ Soak the gelatin in the honey and water. Dissolve over low heat and add the glycerin. Cool to lukewarm, and add the oil of lavender.

GLYCERIN JELLY [1]

Gelatin	1 teaspoon
Glycerin	2 tablespoons
Alcohol	1 teaspoon
Water	1/4 cup

☞ Soak the gelatin in the water to soften it. Dissolve over low heat. Cool to lukewarm before adding the other ingredients.

GLYCERIN JELLY [2]

Gelatin	1 tablespoon
Boric acid powder	1 tablespoon
Glycerin	3/4 cup
Water	1 1/4 cups

☞ Soften the gelatin in the water, then dissolve over low heat. Add the boric acid, and stir until dissolved. Add the glycerin.

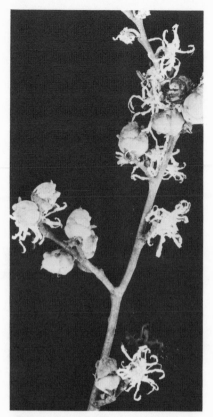 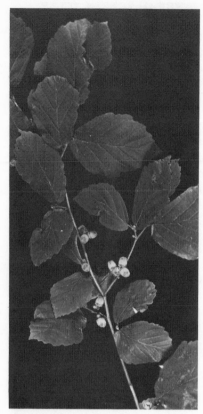

Witch hazel, a small tree, was used by the Indians and is still used as an astringent in shaving lotions. Left, blossoms; right, fruits and leaves. (Hamamelis virginiana) U.S. Forest Service.

PETROLEUM CLEANSING JELLY

Camphor, coarsely powdered	1 teaspoon
Paraffin	1 teaspoon
Glycerin	1 teaspoon
Beeswax	2 tablespoons
Petroleum jelly	1/2 cup

☞ Melt the paraffin, petroleum jelly, and wax together. Stir in the camphor and glycerin.

QUINCE SEED JELLY

Quince seeds	2 teaspoons
Borax	1 teaspoon

Cologne water	1 tablespoon
Glycerin	1/4 cup
Water, hot	1 1/4 cups

☛ Soak the quince seeds in the water to form a mucilage. Strain, then add the remaining ingredients.

TRAGACANTH CLEANSING JELLY

Tragacanth	2 teaspoons
Borax	1 teaspoon
Glycerin	1/4 cup
Water	1 1/2 cups

☛ Soak the tragacanth in the water to form a mucilage. Dissolve the borax in the glycerin, and combine with the mucilage.

WITCH HAZEL JELLY

Gelatin	1 tablespoon
Glycerin	2 tablespoons
Witch hazel	1 cup

☛ Soften the gelatin in the witch hazel. Dissolve over a water bath, and add the glycerin.

CLEANSING CREAMS

ALMOND CLEANSING CREAM [1]

Almonds, sliced	1/4 cup
Almond oil	2 teaspoons
Quince seeds	2 teaspoons
Borax	1 teaspoon
Alcohol	2 tablespoons
Water, hot	1 cup
Oil of rose	8 drops

☛ Combine the almonds, alcohol, and almond oil in a blender. Add the quince seeds to the water, and let set to form a mucilage. Strain the mucilage, and add to the first mixture. Stir in the borax and oil of rose.

ALMOND CLEANSING CREAM [2]

Almond oil	1 cup
Honey	1 tablespoon
Liquid soap	1/4 teaspoon
Oil of sweet almonds	1/4 teaspoon
Oil of bergamot	1/4 teaspoon

☞ Combine the honey and almond oil. Stir in the soap and the scented oils.

ALMOND-GLYCERIN CLEANSING CREAM

Soap flakes	1 teaspoon
Boric acid powder	2 teaspoons
Tragacanth	2 teaspoons
Glycerin	1/4 cup
Water, hot	1 1/2 cups
Oil of bitter almonds	10 drops

☞ Soak the tragacanth in the water to form a mucilage. Stir in the remaining ingredients.

ALMOND-ROSE CLEANSING CREAM [1]

Almonds, sliced	1/2 cup
Borax	1 teaspoon
Glycerin	1/4 cup
Cologne water	1 teaspoon (see Chapter 6, Colognes)
Rosewater	1/2 cup

☞ Combine the almonds and rosewater in a blender. Add the remaining ingredients.

ALMOND-ROSE CLEANSING CREAM [2]

Almonds, sliced	1/2 cup
Borax	1/2 teaspoon

Tincture of benzoin	1 teaspoon
Glycerin	1 1/2 tablespoons
Rosewater	1 cup

☞ Combine the almonds and rosewater in a blender. Add the remaining ingredients.

EGG CLEANSING CREAM

Gum acacia	1 1/2 teaspoons
Honey	3 tablespoons
Egg yolk	1
Liquid soap	1 teaspoon
Olive oil	1 cup
Oil of lemon	1 teaspoon

☞ Mix the acacia, honey, and egg yolk together into a smooth paste. Combine the soap, olive oil, and oil of lemon, and stir gradually into the honey mixture.

ELDER-FLOWER CLEANSING CREAM

| Elder-flower water | 1/2 cup |
| Glycerin | 1/2 cup |

☞ Combine ingredients.

GLYCERIN CLEANSING CREAM [1]

Tragacanth	1 1/2 teaspoons
Glycerin	1 tablespoon
Camphor	1/2 teaspoon
Water	1 cup

☞ Soak the tragacanth in the water to form a mucilage. Add the glycerin and camphor.

GLYCERIN CLEANSING CREAM [2]

Quince seed	2 teaspoons
Water, hot	1 3/4 cups
Borax	1 teaspoon
Glycerin	1/4 cup
Camphor	1/4 teaspoon
Alcohol	2 tablespoons
Oil of bitter almond	10 drops

☛ Soak the quince seed in the water to form a mucilage. Strain, then add the glycerin and the borax. Dissolve the oil and camphor in the alcohol, and add to the first mixture.

GLYCERIN CLEANSING CREAM [3]

Tragacanth	1 teaspoon
Alcohol	1/4 cup
Water, hot	1 1/2 cups
Glycerin	1/2 cup

☛ Soak the tragacanth in the water to form a mucilage. Add the alcohol and glycerin.

GLYCERIN-ALMOND CLEANSING CREAM

Almond oil	1 cup
Glycerin	1/4 cup
Beeswax	1/4 cup
Liquid soap	1 tablespoon
Oil of rose	10 drops
Oil of lemon	1/8 teaspoon

☛ Melt the wax with the almond oil over low heat. Combine the soap, glycerin, and perfume oils. Stir this mixture gradually into the almond oil mixture, and heat until a smooth cream is formed.

GLYCERIN–ORANGE-FLOWER WATER CLEANSING CREAM

Cologne water	2 tablespoons
Orange-flower water	3 tablespoons
Glycerin	1/2 cup

☛ Combine ingredients.

GLYCERIN-CORNSTARCH CLEANSING CREAM

Cornstarch	2 tablespoons
Water	1/4 cup
Glycerin	1/4 cup
Oil of bay	1/8 teaspoon
Alcohol	1 tablespoon

☛ Combine the cornstarch, water, and glycerin. Heat, stirring constantly, until a smooth paste is formed. Let cool and add the oil of bay and alcohol.

HONEY CLEANSING CREAM

Liquid soap	1 1/2 tablespoons
Honey	1/4 cup
Rosewater	1/2 cup

☛ Combine ingredients.

HONEY AND ALMOND CLEANSING CREAM

Almond oil	1 teaspoon
Glycerin	1 teaspoon
Cold cream, commercial	1 teaspoon
Boric acid powder	1/2 teaspoon
Quince seed	1 teaspoon
Water, hot	1 cup

☛ Combine the quince seed and water, and let set to form a mucilage. Strain, then add the remaining ingredients.

IRISH MOSS CLEANSING CREAM [1]

Irish moss	2 teaspoons
Water	1 1/4 cups
Glycerin	1/4 cup
Boric acid powder	1/2 teaspoon
Cologne water	2 tablespoons

☛ Boil the Irish moss with the water to form a mucilage. Add the boric acid and glycerin. Let cool, and add the cologne water.

IRISH MOSS CLEANSING CREAM [2]

Irish moss	1 1/2 teaspoons
Glycerin	1 tablespoon
Alcohol	2 tablespoons
Boric acid powder	1/2 teaspoon
Water	1 cup

☞ Boil the Irish moss with the water to form a mucilage. Add the remaining ingredients.

JASMINE CLEANSING CREAM

Tragacanth	1 1/2 teaspoons
Borax	1 teaspoon
Glycerin	1/2 cup
Oil of jasmine	1/8 teaspoon
Rosewater	1/2 cup
Water, hot	1/2 cup
Alcohol	1 1/2 tablespoons

☞ Soak the tragacanth in the water to form a mucilage. Combine the remaining ingredients and add to the mucilage.

LANOLIN-COCONUT CLEANSING CREAM

Lanolin	1/2 cup
Coconut oil	1/4 cup plus 2 tablespoons
Water	1/4 cup

☞ Melt the lanolin over low heat. Stir in the coconut oil, then add the water.

LANOLIN CLEANSING CREAM [1]

Lanolin	3/4 cup
Sunflower oil	1/4 cup
Water	3 tablespoons

☞ Melt the lanolin over low heat. Stir in the sunflower oil, then add the water gradually.

LANOLIN CLEANSING CREAM [2]

Petroleum jelly	1 cup
Paraffin	1/4 cup
Lanolin	2 tablespoons
Water	1/3 cup
Oil of rose	5 drops
Vanilla extract	1 teaspoon

☛ Melt the wax and petroleum jelly over low heat. Stir in the lanolin, then add the water gradually. Add the remaining ingredients.

LILY CLEANSING CREAM

Carob bean powder	1 1/2 tablespoons
Glycerin	1/2 cup
Water	1 cup
Lily-scented cologne	1 teaspoon
Alcohol	1 tablespoon
Tincture of benzoin	1/2 teaspoon

☛ Soak the carob bean powder in the water to form a mucilage. Combine the glycerin, cologne, and alcohol, and add to the mucilage. Stir in the tincture of benzoin.

LINSEED CLEANSING CREAM

Linseed	1 1/2 teaspoons
Boric acid powder	1/2 teaspoon
Glycerin	2 tablespoons
Alcohol	1/4 cup
Water	1 cup

☛ Bring the water and linseed to a boil, and simmer until a mucilage is formed. Strain, and add the boric acid, glycerin, and alcohol.

LOCUST BEAN CLEANSING CREAM

Locust bean gum	1 teaspoon
Glycerin	1/4 cup
Water	1/2 cup
Alcohol	2 teaspoons
Boric acid powder	1/2 teaspoon

☞ Soak the locust bean gum in the water to form a mucilage. Stir in the remaining ingredients.

MENTHOL CLEANSING CREAM

Tragacanth	2 teaspoons
Glycerin	1 tablespoon
Menthol	1/2 teaspoon
Alcohol	2 tablespoons
Water, hot	1 3/4 cups

☞ Soak the tragacanth in the water to form a mucilage. Dissolve the menthol in the alcohol, and add the glycerin. Combine the two mixtures.

MILKMAID CLEANSING CREAM

Glycerin	1/4 cup
Petroleum jelly	2 tablespoons
Lanolin	1/4 cup
Oil of lemon	9 drops

☞ Melt the lanolin and the petroleum jelly over low heat. Stir in the remaining ingredients.

OLIVE OIL CLEANSING CREAM

Olive oil	1/4 cup
Petroleum jelly	1/4 cup
Borax	1/2 teaspoon

☞ Melt the petroleum jelly over low heat. Stir in the olive oil and borax.

ORANGE-FLOWER CLEANSING CREAM

Cornstarch	2 tablespoons
Irish moss	1 teaspoon
Boric acid powder	1 1/2 teaspoons
Glycerin	1/4 cup
Orange-flower water	3/4 cup
Water	1 cup

☛ Boil the Irish moss with the water to form a mucilage. Add the starch, boric acid, and glycerin, and stir until smooth. Stir in the orange-flower water.

QUINCE SEED CLEANSING CREAM [1]

Quince seed	1 1/2 teaspoons
Borax	1 teaspoon
Glycerin	1/4 cup
Water, hot	3/4 cup
Cologne water	2 tablespoons

☛ Combine the quince seed and water, and let set to form a mucilage. Strain, then add the glycerin and borax. Stir in the cologne water.

QUINCE SEED CLEANSING CREAM [2]

Quince seed	2 teaspoons
Borax	1 teaspoon
Boric acid powder	1 teaspoon
Glycerin	1/4 cup
Alcohol	1/4 cup
Water, hot	1 1/2 cups

☛ Combine the quince seed and water, and let set to form a mucilage. Strain, then add the alcohol, borax, and boric acid. Stir in the glycerin.

ROSE CLEANSING CREAM [1]

Almonds, sliced	1/4 cup
Almond oil	1 teaspoon
Liquid soap	1 teaspoon
Rosewater	1 cup

☞ Combine the almonds with the rosewater in a blender. Add the almond oil and soap.

ROSE CLEANSING CREAM [2]

Borax	2 tablespoons
Tincture of benzoin	1 teaspoon
Glycerin	2 tablespoons
Alcohol	2 tablespoons
Rosewater	1/2 cup

☞ Dissolve the borax in the rosewater. Add the remaining ingredients.

ROSE CLEANSING CREAM [3]

Cornstarch	2 tablespoons
Irish moss	1/2 teaspoon
Boric acid powder	1 teaspoon
Glycerin	1/4 cup
Rosewater	3/4 cup
Water	1 cup

☞ Boil the Irish moss with the water to form a mucilage. Add the cornstarch and boric acid, stirring over low heat until a smooth paste is formed. Add the glycerin and the rosewater.

SESAME OIL CLEANSING CREAM

Soap flakes	1/4 cup
Sesame oil	1 tablespoon

Oil of orange	1/2 teaspoon
Water, hot	1 cup

☞ Dissolve the soap in the water. Add the sesame oil and oil of orange.

STRAWBERRY CLEANSING CREAM

Almond oil	1 1/2 teaspoons
Glycerin	1 1/2 teaspoons
Gum arabic	1 1/2 teaspoons
Water	1 1/2 cups
Tincture of benzoin	1 tablespoon
Oil of strawberry	2 teaspoons

☞ Soak the gum arabic in the water to form a mucilage. Add the almond oil and the glycerin, and shake well. Add the tincture of benzoin and the oil of strawberry.

TALC CLEANSING CREAM

Talc	1/4 cup
Glycerin	1/4 cup
Boric acid powder	1/2 teaspoon
Cologne water	1/4 cup
Water	2 cups

☞ Mix the talc with 1/4 cup of water until a smooth mixture is formed. Add the rest of the water, and stir over low heat until the mixture becomes clear. Add the glycerin, boric acid, and cologne water.

LAVENDER-TRAGACANTH CLEANSING CREAM

Tragacanth	1/2 teaspoon
Glycerin	1 tablespoon
Water, hot	1/2 cup
Oil of lavender	1/8 teaspoon

☞ Combine the tragacanth and water, and let set to form a mucilage. Stir in the glycerin and the oil.

LEMON-TRAGACANTH CLEANSING CREAM

Tragacanth	1 teaspoon
Alcohol	2 tablespoons
Glycerin	1 tablespoon
Water, hot	1 cup
Oil of lemon	1/4 teaspoon

☛ Combine the tragacanth and the water, and let set to form a mucilage. Add the remaining ingredients.

LIME-TRAGACANTH CLEANSING CREAM

Tragacanth	1 teaspoon
Water, hot	1 cup
Glycerin	1 tablespoon
Tincture of benzoin	2 teaspoons
Borax	1/4 teaspoon
Oil of lime	1/8 teaspoon

☛ Soak the tragacanth in the water to form a mucilage. Dissolve the borax and oil of lime in the tincture of benzoin, and add to the mucilage. Stir in the glycerin.

TRAGACANTH CLEANSING CREAM [1]

Tragacanth	2 teaspoons
Boric acid powder	1/2 teaspoon
Glycerin	1/4 cup
Alcohol	1/4 cup
Water, hot	1 1/2 cups

☛ Soak the tragacanth in the water to form a mucilage. Add the glycerin, boric acid, and alcohol.

TRAGACANTH CLEANSING CREAM [2]

Tragacanth	2 teaspoons
Alcohol	1/4 cup

| Glycerin | 1/4 cup |
| Water, hot | 1 1/2 cups |

☛ Combine the tragacanth and water, and let set to form a mucilage. Add the glycerin and alcohol.

WITCH HAZEL CLEANSING CREAM [1]

Quince seed	1 teaspoon
Borax	1/2 teaspoon
Glycerin	1 tablespoon
Alcohol	1 tablespoon
Water, hot	1/4 cup
Witch hazel	1 cup

☛ Combine the quince seed and water, and let set to form a mucilage. Strain, then add the remaining ingredients.

WITCH HAZEL CLEANSING CREAM [2]

Glycerin	2 tablespoons
Quince seed	1 teaspoon
Water, hot	1/2 cup
Witch hazel	2 tablespoons
Alcohol	2 tablespoons

☛ Combine the quince seed and the water, and let set to form a mucilage. Strain, and add the remaining ingredients.

CLEANSING ICES

CAMPHOR CLEANSING ICE

Petroleum jelly	1/2 cup
Paraffin	5 tablespoons
Camphor	1 tablespoon

☛ Melt the petroleum jelly and the paraffin together over low heat. Add the camphor and stir until dissolved.

PETROLEUM JELLY CLEANSING ICE

Camphor	1 teaspoon
Paraffin	1/4 cup
Glycerin	1 tablespoon
Beeswax	1/2 cup
Petroleum jelly	1/2 cup

☞ Melt the paraffin, beeswax, and petroleum jelly together over low heat. Add the camphor, and stir until dissolved. Stir in the glycerin.

COLD CREAMS

ALMOND COLD CREAM [1]

Beeswax	1 tablespoon
Almond oil	1/2 cup
Water	1/4 cup
Borax	1 teaspoon

☞ Melt the beeswax over low heat. Add the almond oil and the borax. Pour into the water in a steady stream, stirring constantly. Continue stirring until the mixture becomes cold.

ALMOND COLD CREAM [2]

Beeswax	2 tablespoons
Petroleum jelly	1 1/2 tablespoons
Mineral oil	1/4 cup
Water, hot	1 1/2 tablespoons
Boric acid powder	1/2 teaspoon
Oil of bitter almond	1 teaspoon

☞ Melt the wax and the petroleum jelly together. Add the mineral oil. Dissolve the boric acid in the water and stir gradually into the wax mixture. Add the oil of bitter almond.

ROSE-ALMOND COLD CREAM

Petroleum jelly	1/2 cup
Beeswax	1/2 cup
Almond oil	1/2 cup
Borax	1 teaspoon
Rosewater	1/4 cup
Oil of rose	10 drops

☞ Melt the petroleum jelly and beeswax over low heat. Stir in the almond oil and borax. Add the rosewater in a steady stream, stirring constantly. Stir in the oil of rose, and continue stirring until the mixture becomes cold.

COTTONSEED COLD CREAM

Petroleum jelly	1 cup
Beeswax	1/2 cup
Cottonseed oil	2 tablespoons
Rosewater	2 tablespoons

☞ Melt the petroleum jelly and wax together over low heat. Stir in the cottonseed oil. Add the rosewater in a steady stream, stirring constantly. Continue stirring until the mixture stiffens.

CUCUMBER COLD CREAM

Lanolin	1 cup
Almond oil	1/4 cup
Cucumbers	2
Water, hot	1 1/2 cups

☞ Pour the water over the sliced, unpeeled cucumbers. When they become pulpy, squeeze through muslin to remove the juice. Melt the lanolin over low heat. Stir in the almond oil. Add the cucumber juice to the lanolin mixture in a steady stream, stirring constantly.

IRISH MOSS COLD CREAM

Irish moss	2 teaspoons
Borax	1 teaspoon
Glycerin	3/4 cup
Cologne water	1/4 cup
Water	1 cup

☛ Boil the Irish moss with the water to form a mucilage. Stir in the borax and glycerin, and let cool. Add the cologne water.

MENTHOLATED COLD CREAM

Petroleum jelly	1/2 cup plus 1 tablespoon
Beeswax	1/3 cup
Menthol	1/2 teaspoon
Camphor	1/2 teaspoon
Thymol	1/2 teaspoon
Boric acid powder	1 teaspoon

☛ Melt the petroleum jelly and wax together over low heat. Add the other ingredients and stir until the mixture is smooth and thick.

ROSE COLD CREAM

Beeswax	2 tablespoons
Almond oil	1/2 cup
Borax	1 1/2 teaspoons
Rosewater	2 tablespoons

☛ Melt the wax over low heat, then add the almond oil and borax. Add the rosewater in a steady stream, while stirring. Continue stirring until the mixture cools.

SUNFLOWER COLD CREAM

Beeswax	1/3 cup
Petroleum jelly	2 tablespoons
Sunflower oil	1/2 cup

| Rosewater | 1/4 cup |
| Borax | 1 teaspoon |

☛ Melt the beeswax and the petroleum jelly together over low heat. Add the sunflower oil and the borax. Pour in the rosewater, in a steady stream, stirring constantly.

VANILLA COLD CREAM

Petroleum jelly	1/2 cup
Paraffin	2 tablespoons
Lanolin	3 tablespoons
Water	1/4 cup
Vanilla extract	1/2 teaspoon
Oil of rose	5 drops

☛ Melt the petroleum jelly and paraffin together over low heat. Add the lanolin. Pour in the water, in a steady stream, while stirring. Continue stirring until the mixture cools. Add the vanilla extract and the oil of rose.

WALNUT COLD CREAM

Petroleum jelly	2 tablespoons
Lanolin	1 teaspoon
Mineral oil	1/2 cup
Walnut oil	2 tablespoons

☛ Melt the petroleum jelly and lanolin together over low heat. Add the mineral and walnut oils.

COLD CREAM WITH LANOLIN

Beeswax	1/3 cup
Lanolin	1/3 cup
Rendered fat	3/4 cup
Borax	1 teaspoon
Water	1/2 cup

☛ Melt the beeswax and fat together over low heat. Stir in the borax and the lanolin. Add the water in a steady stream, stirring constantly. Continue stirring until the mixture cools.

COLD CREAM [1]

Mineral oil	1/2 cup
Paraffin	1 1/2 tablespoons
Beeswax	1/4 cup
Boric acid powder	1 teaspoon
Water, hot	1/2 cup

☛ Melt the wax, paraffin, and mineral oil together over low heat. Add the boric acid. Stir while adding the water in a steady stream.

COLD CREAM [2]

Lanolin	1 tablespoon
Mineral oil	1/4 cup
Petroleum jelly	2 tablespoons
Water	1/3 cup

☛ Melt the lanolin and petroleum jelly together. Add the mineral oil. Stir while adding the water gradually in a steady stream.

COLD CREAM [3]

Beeswax	2 tablespoons
Mineral oil	1/2 cup
Water	1/4 cup
Boric acid powder	1 teaspoon

☛ Melt the beeswax over low heat. Stir in the mineral oil and the boric acid. While stirring, add the water gradually in a steady stream.

Colognes & Perfumes

Modern colognes and perfumes are very similar in composition, differing mainly in the strength of the alcohol and in the amount of the aromatic oil used. Colognes and toilet waters are solutions of 1 to 2 percent aromatic oil, dissolved in 60 to 70 percent alcohol. Perfumes vary in their aromatic oil content from 4–5 percent to as high as 20 percent or more, dissolved in 95 percent alcohol.

In the Old Testament, Exodus 3:23–24, reference is made to the religious objects of the synagogue, including olive oil, cassia, calamus, myrrh, and cinnamon. The Egyptians used sweet-smelling sachets, aromatic incense, and scented powders for perfumes. Ultimately they learned to extract aromatic oil from plants by steeping them in different fats, oils, or wines.

Probably the most popular aromatic oil used is otto of rose. A lovely legend has it that an *Arabian Nights* princess living in Persia noticed oil floating in a castle moat into which roses had fallen. She had her servants skim off the oil and found it to be pleasant and refreshing.

Perfumes were made and sold in Paris in the early 1200s but were not commonly used in England. Most early European perfumes were in the form of dried plants carried in small cloth or silk bags, or in tiny bottles enclosed in some piece of jewelry, or sprinkled on linens. Rose petals were featured in almost all, as were gums and often violets.

Colognes, offspring of perfume, were the creation of an Italian nobleman-botanist, Frangipane, who accompanied Columbus on one of his voyages, and had the lovely West Indian tropical flower, frangipani, named after him. If history is dependable in this case, the good botanist found that by putting dried aromatic flowers in white wine he had a perfume that persisted longer than the original dry perfumes.

After this discovery, a wave of "colognes" spread over Europe, including eau de cologne, Hungary water, and lavender water. These were, for the most part, made by distilling different herbs and flowers in water.

Colognes are usually less expensive than perfumes because they contain less of the aromatic oils. Only two perfume formulas are given

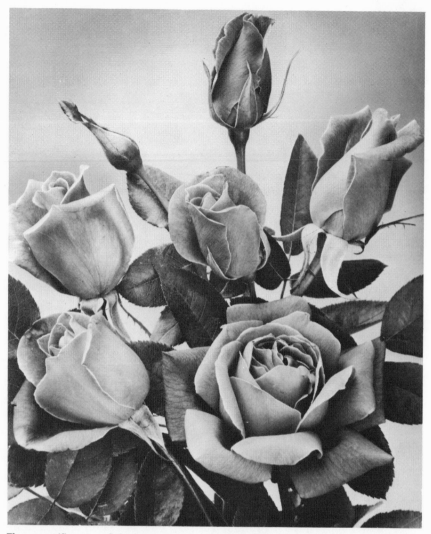

**The magnificent and fragrant rose is undoubtedly the queen of cosmetic ingre-
dients, as it has been from the time of ancient Rome and Greece.** U.S. Department of Agriculture.

in this section because making perfumes is very expensive. (The user
of this guide can, of course, design his own perfume formulas.)

When no instructions are given in the following formulas, the ingredients are merely combined. Bear in mind also that it may be
necessary to age these colognes and perfumes for a week or more, so
that the different aromas may blend and absorb the natural smell of
the alcohol.

COLOGNE WATER

COLOGNE WATER [1]

Alcohol (60 percent)	2 cups
Oil of lemon	1/8 teaspoon
Oil of bergamot	1 tablespoon
Oil of lavender	1/8 teaspoon

COLOGNE WATER [2]

Alcohol (60 percent)	2 cups
Oil of lemon	1 1/2 teaspoons
Oil of bergamot	1/8 teaspoon
Oil of neroli	1/4 teaspoon
Oil of lavender	1/8 teaspoon
Oil of rosemary	10 drops

COLOGNE WATER [3]

Alcohol (60 percent)	1 1/2 cups
Oil of orange	2 tablespoons
Oil of lemon	2 tablespoons
Oil of bergamot	1 tablespoon
Oil of rose	3 drops
Water	1/3 cup

☞ Dissolve the oils in the alcohol. Add the water.

COLOGNE WATER [4]

Alcohol (60 percent)	2 cups
Oil of lemon	1/2 teaspoon
Oil of neroli	7 drops
Oil of bergamot	1 1/2 teaspoon
Oil of melissa	7 drops
Oil of lavender	1/4 teaspoon

COLOGNE WATER [5]

Alcohol (60 percent)	1 3/4 cup plus 2 tablespoons
Oil of bergamot	1 1/2 teaspoons
Oil of lemon	16 drops
Oil of lavender	8 drops
Oil of melissa	1/4 teaspoon
Oil of neroli	8 drops

COLOGNE WATER [6]

Alcohol (60 percent)	2 cups
Oil of bergamot	1/8 teaspoon
Oil of lemon	1 1/2 teaspoons
Oil of lavender	1/8 teaspoon
Oil of rosemary	1/8 teaspoon
Oil of cloves	5 drops

COLOGNE WATER [7]

Alcohol (60 percent)	2 cups
Oil of orange	1/8 teaspoon
Oil of bergamot	1/4 teaspoon
Oil of citron	1/8 teaspoon
Oil of rosemary	1/4 teaspoon
Oil of neroli	1/2 teaspoon

COLOGNE WATER [8]

Alcohol (60 percent)	1 1/2 cups
Oil of orange	2 tablespoons
Oil of bergamot	1/4 teaspoon
Oil of lemon	1 tablespoon
Oil of rose	10 drops
Water	1/4 cup plus 1 tablespoon

☛ Dissolve the oils in the alcohol. Add the water.

COLOGNE WATER [9]

Alcohol (60 percent)	1 3/4 cups
Tincture of benzoin	1/8 teaspoon
Oil of orange	1/8 teaspoon
Oil of bergamot	1/8 teaspoon
Oil of lemon	1/4 teaspoon
Oil of rosemary	1/8 teaspoon
Oil of neroli	1/4 teaspoon
Orange-flower water	3 tablespoons

☞ Dissolve the oils in the alcohol. Add the tincture of benzoin, and then gradually add the orange flower water.

COLOGNE WATER [10]

Alcohol (60 percent)	1 3/4 cups
Oil of neroli	1/8 teaspoon
Oil of bergamot	1/8 teaspoon
Oil of rosemary	10 drops
Extract of jasmine	1/2 teaspoon
Water	1/4 cup

☞ Dissolve the oils in the alcohol. Add the extract of jasmine. Add the water gradually.

FLORIDA WATERS

FLORIDA WATER

Alcohol (60 percent)	2 cups
Oil of lavender	1 teaspoon
Oil of bergamot	1 1/2 teaspoons
Oil of lemon	1/4 teaspoon
Oil of cloves	1/2 teaspoon

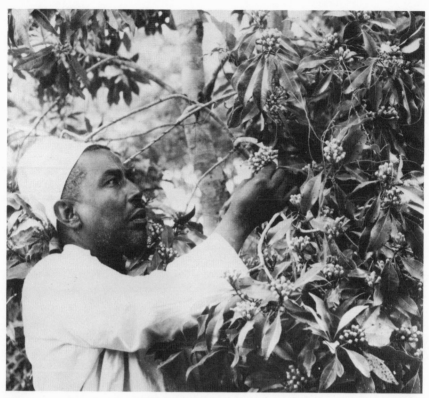

Cloves, common in most kitchens, are also used in sachets and as flavoring in toothpastes and mouth washes. Oil of cloves is used in bath preparations and colognes. The photo shows the harvesting of the unopened buds of the clove tree in Zanzibar, the world's center of cloves. (Syzygium aromaticum) American Spice Trade Association.

LEMON-GRASS FLORIDA WATER

Alcohol (60 percent)	1 1/2 cups
Oil of lavender	1 1/2 teaspoons
Oil of lemon	3/4 teaspoon
Oil of lemon grass	1/4 teaspoon
Oil of cloves	1/2 teaspoon
Water	1/2 cup

☞ Dissolve the oils in the alcohol, then add the water.

MINT FLORIDA WATER

Alcohol (60 percent)	3/4 cup
Oil of lavender	1 teaspoon

Oil of cloves	1/8 teaspoon
Oil of bergamot	15 drops
Oil of rose geranium	1/8 teaspoon
Oil of spearmint	7 drops
Benzoic acid	1/8 teaspoon
Water	2 tablespoons

☞ Dissolve the oils in the alcohol. Add the benzoic acid, and then the water.

ROSE FLORIDA WATER

Alcohol (60 percent)	1 1/3 cups
Oil of lavender	1 1/2 teaspoons
Oil of lemon	1/4 teaspoon
Oil of lemon grass	1/2 teaspoon
Oil of cloves	1 teaspoon
Rosewater	1/2 cup plus 2 tablespoons

☞ Dissolve the oils in the alcohol, then add the rosewater.

HUNGARY WATERS

HUNGARY WATER

Alcohol (60 percent)	1 3/4 cups
Oil of rosemary	1 1/2 teaspoons
Oil of lemon	3/4 teaspoon
Spirit of rose	1/4 cup

MAGYAR HUNGARY WATER

Alcohol (60 percent)	1 3/4 cups
Oil of rosemary	2 teaspoons
Oil of melissa	1 teaspoon
Oil of lemon	1 teaspoon
Oil of peppermint	3 drops
Extract of neroli	2 tablespoons
Extract of rose	2 tablespoons

☞ Dissolve the oils in the alcohol. Add the extracts.

ST. STEPHAN'S HUNGARY WATER

Alcohol (60 percent)	1 1/2 cups plus 2 tablespoons
Oil of lemon	1/8 teaspoon
Oil of melissa	1/8 teaspoon
Oil of rosemary	1 1/2 teaspoons
Oil of peppermint	10 drops
Extract of rose	3 tablespoons
Extract of neroli	3 tablespoons

☞ Dissolve the oils in the alcohol, then add the extracts.

OTHER WATERS

LAVENDER WATER

Alcohol (60 percent)	1 1/2 cups
Oil of lavender	1 1/2 teaspoons
Rosewater	1/2 cup

☞ Dissolve the oil in the alcohol, then add the rosewater.

LEMON VERBENA WATER

Alcohol (60 percent)	1/2 cup plus 1 tablespoon
Tincture of orris	1 tablespoon
Spirit of lemon	1 cup plus 1 tablespoon
Spirit of lemon grass	1/4 cup plus 1 tablespoon

LILAC WATER

Alcohol (60 percent)	1 3/4 cups plus 1 tablespoon
Tincture of benzoin	1/2 teaspoon
Oil of orange	1/4 teaspoon
Oil of lemon	1/4 teaspoon

Oil of bergamot	1/8 teaspoon
Oil of rosemary	1/4 teaspoon
Terpineol	1/8 teaspoon
Water	3 tablespoons

☞ Dissolve the oils in the alcohol. Add the tincture of benzoin and the terpineol. Shake well and add the water.

ORANGE VERBENA WATER

Alcohol (60 percent)	1 1/2 cups plus 2 tablespoons
Tincture of orris	1 1/2 tablespoons
Extract of jasmine	1/4 teaspoon
Oil of verbena	1/8 teaspoon
Oil of orange	1/8 teaspoon
Oil of lemon	1/8 teaspoon
Oil of neroli	5 drops
Rosewater	3 tablespoons

☞ Dissolve the oils in the alcohol. Add the extract of jasmine and the tincture of orris. Shake well and add the rosewater.

VIOLET WATER

Alcohol (60 percent)	1 1/2 cups plus 2 tablespoons
Extract of orris	1/4 cup
Extract of cassie	1 tablespoon
Extract of rose	1 tablespoon

ALMOND-VIOLET WATER

Alcohol (60 percent)	3 tablespoons
Tincture of orris	1/4 cup
Spirit of almond	1 tablespoon
Extract of cassie	1/4 cup plus 2 tablespoons
Extract of rose	5 tablespoons
Extract of tuberose	1/3 cup

CASSIE-VIOLET WATER

Alcohol (60 percent)	1 1/2 cups plus 3 tablespoons
Spirit of rose	1 tablespoon
Extract of orris	3 tablespoons
Extract of cassie	1 tablespoon

COLOGNES

BAVARIAN COLOGNE

Alcohol (60 percent)	1 3/4 cups
Oil of sandalwood	1/4 teaspoon
Oil of lemon	1/8 teaspoon
Oil of bergamot	1/8 teaspoon
Oil of neroli	17 drops
Camphor	1/8 teaspoon

☞ Dissolve the camphor in the alcohol and add the oils.

BAY RUM COLOGNE

Oil of bay	1/2 teaspoon
Tincture of bay leaves	1/2 cup plus 2 tablespoons

PUERTO RICAN BAY RUM COLOGNE

Alcohol (60 percent)	1/2 cup plus 2 tablespoons
Oil of bay	1 tablespoon
Oil of pimento	3 drops

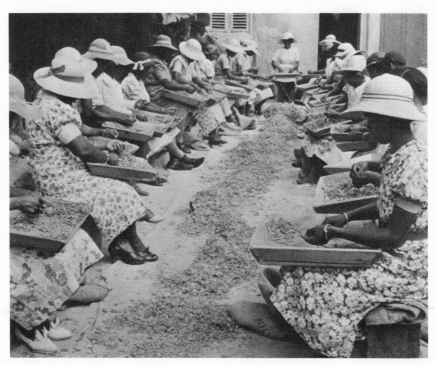

Mace and nutmeg come from the same tropical fruit. Their oil is used in colognes, sachets, mouth washes, and toothpastes. In the photo, West Indian women are removing the mace, a lacy material which surrounds the nutmeg. (Myristica fragrans) American Spice Trade Association.

Oil of rose	4 drops
Rum	2 tablespoons
Water	1 1/4 cups

☞ Dissolve the oils in the alcohol, then add the rum and water.

VIRGIN ISLANDS BAY RUM COLOGNE

Alcohol (60 percent)	1 1/4 cups
Oil of bay	1/8 teaspoon
Virgin Islands rum	1 tablespoon
Water	3/4 cup

☞ Dissolve the oil in the alcohol. Add the rum and the water.

WEST INDIES BAY RUM COLOGNE

Alcohol (60 percent)	1 cup
Oil of bay	1/8 teaspoon
Oil of pimento	10 drops
Oil of orange	10 drops
Orrisroot powder	1 1/2 teaspoons
Tincture of benzoin	1/4 teaspoon
Water	1 cup

☞ Dissolve the oils in the alcohol. Add the tincture of benzoin and the orrisroot. Stir in the water gradually. Put through a filter to remove any particles of the orrisroot.

BUTTERFLY COLOGNE

Tincture of tonka bean	1/4 cup
Extract of neroli	3/4 cup
Extract of tuberose	3/4 cup
Extract of rose	1/4 cup

CAROLINA COLOGNE

Alcohol (60 percent)	3/4 cup
Oil of lemon	1/2 teaspoon
Oil of lemon grass	1/4 teaspoon
Oil of lavender	1 teaspoon
Oil of cloves	3 drops
Water	1/4 cup plus 2 tablespoons

☞ Dissolve the oils in the alcohol and add the water.

CASSIE COLOGNE

Spirit of vanilla	1/4 cup
Spirit of neroli	1/2 cup
Spirit of cassie	1/2 cup
Spirit of rose	1 cup
Oil of cloves	10 drops

CELIA'S COLOGNE

Extract of vanilla	1/4 cup plus 2 tablespoons
Extract of neroli	1/4 cup plus 2 tablespoons
Extract of rose	3/4 cup
Extract of cassie	1/4 cup plus 2 tablespoons
Oil of cloves	1/8 teaspoon

COUNTRY GIRL COLOGNE

Alcohol (60 percent)	1 1/4 cups plus 2 tablespoons
Spirit of almond	3/4 cup
Spirit of lemon	3 tablespoons
Extract of peach flowers	1/4 cup plus 2 tablespoons
Extract of tuberose	1 1/2 tablespoons
Peru balsam	1/2 teaspoon

EASTER COLOGNE

Alcohol (60 percent)	2 cups
Tincture of vanilla	3 tablespoons
Tincture of cassie	2 1/2 tablespoons
Spirit of cloves	1 tablespoon
Extract of rose	1/4 cup plus 1 tablespoon
Extract of neroli	2 1/2 tablespoons

ELEAGNUS COLOGNE

Alcohol (60 percent)	1 1/2 cups
Spirit of bergamot	1 tablespoon
Extract of rose	1/4 cup
Extract of cassie	1 tablespoon
Extract of jasmine	3 tablespoons
Extract of orris	3 tablespoons

FLORAL COLOGNE

Alcohol (60 percent)	1 1/2 cups
Tincture of tonka bean	1/4 cup
Extract of neroli	1 1/2 tablespoons
Extract of cassie	1 1/2 tablespoons
Extract of rose	1/4 cup
Oil of citronella	1/4 teaspoon

FLORIDA COLOGNE

Alcohol (60 percent)	2 cups
Oil of orange	1 tablespoon
Oil of lemon	1/8 teaspoon
Oil of rose	10 drops

FLOWERS OF KILLARNEY COLOGNE

Tincture of vanilla	1/4 cup
Extract of rose	1 3/4 cups

GARDENIA COLOGNE

Alcohol (60 percent)	1 3/4 cups
Oil of rose	1/8 teaspoon
Oil of jasmine	10 drops
Oil of sandalwood	10 drops
Oil of bergamot	1/8 teaspoon
Oil of angelica	1 drop
Tincture of vanilla	1/8 teaspoon

HAYRIDE COLOGNE

Tincture of benzoin	1 1/2 teaspoons
Tincture of vanilla	3 tablespoons
Spirit of ambrette	1/4 cup plus 1 tablespoon
Spirit of rose	1/2 cup
Spirit of lavender	2 tablespoons

Extract of jasmine	1/4 cup plus 1 tablespoon
Extract of neroli	1/2 cup
Extract of tuberose	1/4 cup plus 2 tablespoons
Oil of linette	10 drops

LAVINIA'S COLOGNE

Alcohol (60 percent)	1/2 cup
Spirit of bergamot	1/4 cup
Spirit of neroli	2 tablespoons
Spirit of lemon	1/4 cup plus 1 tablespoon
Spirit of lavender	1/4 cup plus 1 tablespoon
Spirit of cloves	1/2 cup

LOUISVILLE COLOGNE

Spirit of neroli	1/4 teaspoon
Spirit of ambrette	2 tablespoons
Extract of jasmine	3 tablespoons
Extract of tuberose	1/2 cup plus 3 tablespoons
Extract of cassie	1/4 cup plus 1 tablespoon

MOONLIGHT COLOGNE

Alcohol (60 percent)	1 1/2 cups
Tincture of tonka bean	2 tablespoons
Spirit of rose	1 tablespoon
Spirit of neroli	1 1/2 tablespoons
Extract of tuberose	2 tablespoons
Extract of neroli	1/2 cup

NEROLI COLOGNE

Tincture of vanilla	1/4 cup
Extract of neroli	1/2 cup
Extract of rose	3/4 cup
Extract of cassie	1/2 cup
Oil of cloves	1/8 teaspoon

NIKO COLOGNE

Tincture of orris	1/4 cup
Extract of verbena	1/4 cup plus 2 tablespoons
Extract of patchouly	1/4 cup plus 3 tablespoons
Extract of sandalwood	1/4 cup
Extract of vetiver	2 tablespoons
Extract of rose	1/4 cup plus 3 tablespoons

PATCHOULY COLOGNE

Alcohol (60 percent)	1 1/4 cups
Spirit of patchouly	3/4 cup
Spirit of rose	1 tablespoon

BERGAMOT-PATCHOULY COLOGNE

Alcohol (60 percent)	1 3/4 cups
Extract of bergamot	1/4 cup
Oil of patchouly	1 1/2 teaspoons
Oil of rose	2 drops

☞ Dissolve the oils in the alcohol. Add the extract.

JASMINE-PATCHOULY COLOGNE

Alcohol (60 percent)	1 1/4 cups plus 1 tablespoon
Tincture of benzoin	1/2 teaspoon
Spirit of bergamot	2 tablespoons
Spirit of patchouly	2 tablespoons
Extract of rose	2 tablespoons
Extract of jasmine	1/4 cup

PLANTATION COLOGNE

Alcohol (60 percent)	1 cup
Oil of bergamot	1/4 teaspoon
Oil of orange	1/4 teaspoon

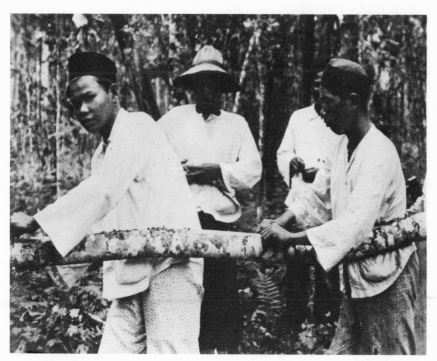

Cinnamon comes from the bark of a tree. Here Indonesians slit the bark and peel off long strips which, as they dry, form the cinnamon sticks we know. This spice is used in colognes, bath preparations, and sachets. (Cinnamomum zeylanicum) American Spice Trade Association.

Oil of lavender	1 teaspoon
Oil of rosemary	1/8 teaspoon
Oil of cinnamon	5 drops

RAMA COLOGNE

Alcohol (60 percent)	1 1/2 cups plus 3 tablespoons
Tincture of sandalwood	1 teaspoon
Extract of rose	1/4 cup plus 1 tablespoon

CLOVE-ROSE COLOGNE

Tincture of vanilla	1/4 cup plus 2 tablespoons
Extract of rose	1 cup plus 2 tablespoons
Extract of neroli	1/2 cup
Oil of cloves	1 1/2 teaspoon

TEA ROSE COLOGNE

Tincture of orris	2 tablespoons
Spirit of sandalwood	1/4 cup
Extract of rose	1 1/2 cups
Extract of neroli	2 tablespoons
Oil of rose geranium	1/4 teaspoon

VIOLET ROSE COLOGNE

Extract of rose	1/2 cup
Extract of orris	1/4 cup
Spirit of patchouly	1/2 tablespoon
Alcohol (60 percent)	1 1/2 cups plus 3 tablespoons
Spirit of jasmine	1/4 cup plus 1 tablespoon

WHITE ROSE COLOGNE

Extract of patchouly	2 tablespoons
Extract of jasmine	1/2 cup
Extract of rose	1 1/2 cups

ROSE COLOGNE

Rosewater	3 tablespoons
Spirit of rose	1/4 cup
Spirit of pimento	2 teaspoons
Spirit of bergamot	3 tablespoons
Spirit of patchouly	1 1/2 tablespoons
Extract of jasmine	1/4 cup plus 1 tablespoon
Alcohol (60 percent)	1 1/4 cups

ROSILLA COLOGNE

Extract of rose	1 cup
Extract of vanilla	1 cup
Oil of bitter almonds	10 drops

SAN PEDRO COLOGNE

Alcohol (60 percent)	2 cups
Oil of neroli	10 drops
Oil of lemon	1 tablespoon
Oil of cloves	1/8 teaspoon
Oil of rose	10 drops

SCOTCH HEATHER COLOGNE

Tincture of orris	1/4 cup plus 2 tablespoons
Extract of vetiver	1/4 cup
Extract of rose	1/4 cup plus 2 tablespoons
Extract of sandalwood	1 cup

SPANISH ISLE COLOGNE

Alcohol (60 percent)	1 3/4 cups plus 2 tablespoons
Oil of orange	1/2 tablespoon
Oil of lemon	1 teaspoon
Oil of rose	8 drops

SPRING COLOGNE

Tincture of tonka bean	1 1/2 cups
Extract of jasmine	1/4 cup
Extract of rose	1/4 cup
Oil of neroli	1/8 teaspoon
Oil of rose	1/8 teaspoon
Oil of rose geranium	1 teaspoon

SPRING FLOWERS COLOGNE

Extract of rose	3/4 cup plus 2 tablespoons
Extract of cassie	2 tablespoons
Extract of orris	3/4 cup
Oil of rose	5 drops
Oil of bergamot	3/4 teaspoon

SWEET COLOGNE

Alcohol (60 percent)	1 3/4 cups
Spirit of almond	1 tablespoon
Spirit of rose	2 tablespoons
Spirit of rose geranium	1/4 cup
Extract of tuberose	1/4 cup plus 3 tablespoons
Extract of neroli	2 tablespoons
Extract of cassie	1/4 cup
Extract of jasmine	1 tablespoon

SWISS COLOGNE

Alcohol (60 percent)	1 1/2 cups plus 3 tablespoons
Oil of orange	5 drops
Oil of lemon	1/2 teaspoon
Oil of neroli	3 drops
Oil of bergamot	1/8 teaspoon
Oil of rosemary	5 drops
Orange-flower water	1/4 cup plus 1 tablespoon

☛ Dissolve the oils in the alcohol, then add the orange-flower water.

TEEKAY COLOGNE

Alcohol (60 percent)	1/4 cup plus 2 tablespoons
Spirit of rose	1/4 cup
Spirit of sandalwood	3/4 cup plus 1 tablespoon
Extract of jasmine	2 tablespoons
Extract of cassie	2 tablespoons
Extract of tuberose	2 tablespoons

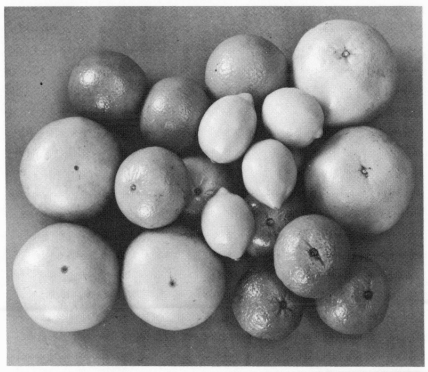

The many kinds of citrus tree are a rich and growing source of scents and essential oils used in a wide range of cosmetics. Dr. W. Grierson, University of Florida, Lake Alfred.

VERBENA COLOGNE

Alcohol (60 percent)	2 cups
Oil of verbena	1 tablespoon
Oil of lemon	1 tablespoon
Oil of neroli	1/2 teaspoon
Oil of rose	1/8 teaspoon
Oil of rose geranium	1 tablespoon

LEMON-VERBENA COLOGNE

Spirit of lemon	1 1/4 cups
Spirit of lemon grass	3/4 cup
Oil of orange	1/4 teaspoon

ROSE-VERBENA COLOGNE

Alcohol (60 percent)	2 cups
Oil of lemon grass	2 1/4 teaspoons
Oil of neroli	1/4 teaspoon
Oil of citron	1 teaspoon
Oil of rose	10 drops
Oil of rose geranium	1 teaspoon

VIOLET COLOGNE

Alcohol (60 percent)	1 1/4 cups
Tincture of orris	1/2 cup
Spirit of almond	1/8 teaspoon
Extract of cassie	2 1/4 teaspoons

ALMOND-VIOLET COLOGNE

Alcohol (60 percent)	1 3/4 cups plus 2 tablespoons
Tincture of orris	1/4 cup
Spirit of almond	1 1/2 teaspoons
Extract of rose	2 tablespoons
Extract of tuberose	2 tablespoons
Extract of cassie	1 1/2 tablespoons

CASSIE-VIOLET COLOGNE

Alcohol (60 percent)	1 cup
Tincture of orris	6 tablespoons
Spirit of rose	1/2 cup
Spirit of almond	1 1/2 teaspoons
Extract of cassie	5 tablespoons
Extract of tuberose	3 tablespoons

ROSE-VIOLET COLOGNE

Extract of orris	1/4 cup
Extract of cassie	3/4 cup
Extract of rose	3/4 cup
Extract of tuberose	1/4 cup

TUBEROSE-VIOLET COLOGNE

Tincture of orris	1/4 cup plus 2 tablespoons
Spirit of almond	2 tablespoons
Extract of cassie	3/4 cup
Extract of rose	1/4 cup plus 2 tablespoons
Extract of tuberose	1/4 cup plus 2 tablespoons

YORK COLOGNE

Alcohol (60 percent)	2 cups
Oil of orange	1/8 teaspoon
Oil of bergamot	1/8 teaspoon
Oil of lavender	1/4 teaspoon
Oil of cinnamon	5 drops
Oil of rosemary	1/8 teaspoon

PERFUMES

DAMASK ROSE PERFUME

Tincture of vanilla	3 tablespoons
Extract of rose	2 cups

ROSE GERANIUM PERFUME

Alcohol (95 percent)	1 3/4 cups plus 2 tablespoons
Oil of rose geranium	2 tablespoons

WHITE ROSE PERFUME

Oil of rose	1/2 teaspoon
Oil of patchouly	1/2 teaspoon
Extract of rose	3/4 cup
Extract of jasmine	3/4 cup
Extract of cassie	1/4 cup plus 2 tablespoons

Complexion Washes

Complexion washes are not so popular now as they once were because ideas of beauty have changed. In medieval Europe a very clear, pale complexion, completely free of all blemishes, freckles, and spots was prized highly as a sign of good breeding. Women went to great lengths to achieve this goal, using highly dangerous washes containing mercury compounds which corroded the skin. Although many famous complexion washes were mixed and sold by traveling magicians and peddlers, women often concocted their own. The ingredients were usually the distilled waters of certain herbs that were believed to bleach the complexion and were, by good fortune, thoroughly harmless.

Today we know the virtues of some of these ingredients. Many of the herbs have been found to be astringent. Egg yolk and honey contain protein and hormones. The acid in citrus fruits does bleach the skin. On the basis of this information, such time-honored washes may still be used effectively, since they do serve as astringents and cleansers.

ANGELICA COMPLEXION WASH

Angelica root, powdered	1 tablespoon
Black hellebore root, powdered	1 tablespoon
Storax	1 1/2 teaspoons
Alcohol	2 cups
Oil of bergamot	10 drops

☛ Add the ingredients to the alcohol and keep for a week in a closed bottle. Strain to remove any undissolved material.

BARLEY COMPLEXION WASH

Barley	1/4 cup
Water	2 cups
Oil of balsam	5 drops

☛ Boil the barley in the water for 10 minutes. Strain, then add the oil to the barley water.

BENZOIN COMPLEXION WASH

Borax	1/2 teaspoon
Tincture of benzoin	1 tablespoon
Water	2 cups

☞ Combine the ingredients.

BENZOIN-ROSE COMPLEXION WASH

Tincture of benzoin	2 teaspoons
Rosewater	2 cups

☞ Combine the ingredients.

DANDELION COMPLEXION WASH

Soap flakes	1 tablespoon
Paraffin	2 tablespoons
Almonds, crushed	2/3 cup
Dandelion juice, fresh	2 tablespoons
Extract of tuberose	1/3 cup
Rosewater	2 cups
Olive oil	1 tablespoon

☞ Melt the soap and paraffin together over low heat. Stir in the almonds and dandelion juice. Strain, and let cool. Add the remaining ingredients.

LAVENDER COMPLEXION WASH

Borax	1/2 teaspoon
Lavender water	1/4 cup
Alcohol	1/2 cup
Tincture of benzoin	1/2 teaspoon
Water	3/4 cup

☞ Combine the ingredients.

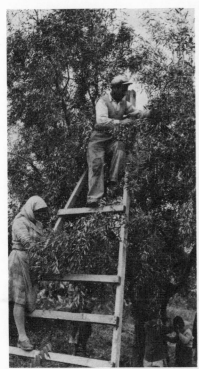 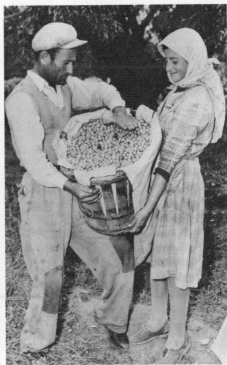

Olive oil is widely used in soaps, bath oils, creams, lotions, and shaving creams. These are scenes in a Greek olive grove at harvesttime. Mutual Security Administration, Greece.

LEMON COMPLEXION WASH

Lemon juice, fresh	1/4 cup
Rosewater	1/4 cup

☞ Combine the ingredients.

ORANGE BLOSSOM COMPLEXION WASH

Potassium carbonate	1/4 cup
Sugar	1 1/2 teaspoons
Orange-flower water	1 1/2 cups
Alcohol	1/4 cup

☞ Combine all the ingredients.

ROSE-ORANGE COMPLEXION WASH

Rosewater	1 cup
Orange-flower water	1/2 cup
Glycerin	1/4 cup
Potassium carbonate	1 teaspoon
Tincture of benzoin	1/2 teaspoon

☞ Combine all the ingredients.

ROSE COMPLEXION WASH

Potassium carbonate	1/4 cup
Water	1 cup
Rosewater	3 tablespoons
Alcohol	2 tablespoons
Oil of rose	10 drops
Oil of cinnamon	1/8 teaspoon

☞ Dissolve the oils in the alcohol. Add the other ingredients and shake well.

SAGE COMPLEXION WASH

Alcohol	1/2 cup
Water	1 cup
Oil of lemon	15 drops
Oil of sage	1/8 teaspoon

☞ Dissolve the oils in the alcohol and add the water.

SPICED COMPLEXION WASH

Fresh lemon peel, sliced	2 tablespoons
Coriander seed	1/4 cup
Ground nutmeg	2 tablespoons
Ground cloves	2 tablespoons
Ground cinnamon	2 tablespoons

| Dried angelica root | 1 tablespoon |
| Alcohol | 2 cups |

☞ Combine all the ingredients. Store in a closed bottle for a week. Strain.

STRAWBERRY COMPLEXION WASH

Strawberries, fresh	1 cup
Alcohol	1 tablespoon
Rosewater	1/4 cup

☞ Puree the strawberries in a blender. Strain and add the juice to the other ingredients.

VIENNA COMPLEXION WASH

Almonds, sliced	1/4 cup
Orange-flower water	1 cup
Rosewater	1/2 cup plus 2 tablespoons
Borax	1 teaspoon
Tincture of benzoin	2 tablespoons

☞ Blend the almonds with the rosewater to make a milk. Add the other ingredients.

BALSAM FRECKLE WASH

Tincture of benzoin	1 teaspoon
Rosewater	2 cups
Balsam	1 teaspoon

☞ Combine the ingredients.

BUTTERMILK FRECKLE WASH

| Buttermilk | 1/4 cup |
| Pomegranate juice | 1/4 teaspoon |

☞ Combine the ingredients.

ELDER-FLOWER FRECKLE WASH

Alum	1 teaspoon
Lemon juice	1 tablespoon
Elder-flower water	3 tablespoons

☞ Combine the ingredients.

ORANGE FLOWER FRECKLE WASH

Potassium carbonate	2 tablespoons
Sugar	1 teaspoon
Orange-flower water	1 3/4 cups
Alcohol	2 tablespoons

☞ Combine the ingredients.

ROSE FRECKLE WASH

Potassium carbonate	2 tablespoons
Water	1 3/4 cups
Rosewater	1 tablespoon
Alcohol	1 tablespoon
Oil of rose	1/8 teaspoon
Oil of cinnamon	1/8 teaspoon

☞ Dissolve the oils in the alcohol. Add the remaining ingredients.

VICIA FABA FRECKLE WASH

Alcohol	1/4 cup
Broad bean (*Vicia faba*) flowers, fresh	1/4 cup
Alum	1 teaspoon
Rosewater	1 cup

☞ Put the flowers in the alcohol in a closed jar overnight. In the morning discard the flowers and add the remaining ingredients.

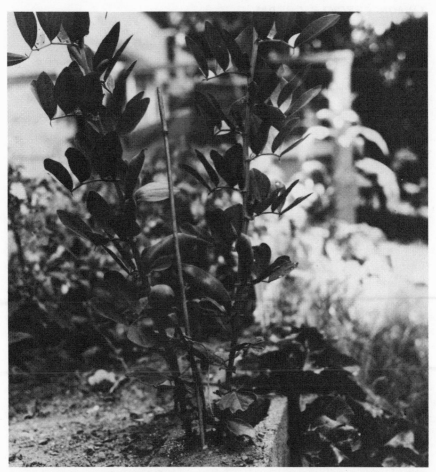

The horse bean is a dietary staple in the Mediterranean basin and has been used in complexion washes for hundreds of years. The beans are sold both dried and canned. (Vicia faba) Arnold Krochmal.

VIENNESE FRECKLE WASH

Rosewater	1 cup
Orange-flower water	1/2 cup
Glycerin	2 tablespoons
Potassium carbonate	2 tablespoons
Tincture of benzoin	1/2 teaspoon

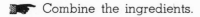 Combine the ingredients.

LEMON FRECKLE CREAM

Apple cider vinegar	1 1/2 cups
The whole lemon, chopped fine	1/4 cup
Alcohol	3 tablespoons
Oil of lavender	1/2 teaspoon
Water	3 tablespoons
Oil of cedarwood	1/4 teaspoon

☛ Soak the lemon in the alcohol overnight. Strain and add the other ingredients. Let set overnight before using.

ORANGE-FLOWER FRECKLE CREAM

Lemon juice	1 tablespoon
Orange-flower water	1 tablespoon
Glycerin	1 tablespoon
Elder flowers, powdered	1 1/2 tablespoons

☛ Combine the ingredients.

VIOLET FRECKLE CREAM

Angelica root powder	2 tablespoons
Orrisroot powder	2 tablespoons
Storax	1/2 teaspoon
Oil of bergamot	1/4 teaspoon
Oil of lemon	1/4 teaspoon
Alcohol	1 cup

☛ Dissolve the oils in the alcohol. Add the remaining ingredients.

BUTTERMILK FRECKLE REMOVER

Buttermilk	1/4 cup
Grated horseradish	1 1/2 teaspoons
Cornmeal	1 1/2 teaspoons

☛ Mix the ingredients and spread the mixture between sheets of soft white cotton. Place the cloth on the face, and leave it there for 10 minutes. After removing it, wash the face with an astringent lotion.

LEMON FRECKLE REMOVER

Whole lemon, chopped	1/4 cup
Oil of lavender	1 1/2 teaspoons
Oil of rose	10 drops
Oil of cedarwood	1/2 teaspoon
Wine vinegar	1 1/2 cups
Alcohol	3 tablespoons
Water	3 tablespoons

☞ Dissolve the oils in the alcohol. Add the other ingredients. Place in a covered jar for three days. Strain to remove the lemon.

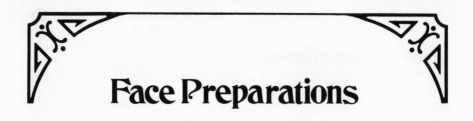

Face Preparations

FACIAL MASKS

The purpose of a facial mask is a general toning of the skin. It is refreshing, closes the pores, and is thought to reduce wrinkles by tightening the skin.

Facial preparations have their origins in antiquity. The Egyptians used egg whites as a facial mask. Roman writers (all men) rebuked women for spending much of the day idly, applying various types of facial masks. Roman matrons used basically the same ingredients as we do now—the different flours of grains and beans, and certain dried plants. The recorded formulas for Roman facials included one made of pea flour and barley meal. This was left on the face for hours, then removed with a milk wash.

Henry III of France used a facial preparation made of egg whites and flour, which was removed with chervil water.

From a practical viewpoint, the facial mask affords the woman user about 20 minutes of complete relaxation and rest, which may do as much for her skin as the ingredients in the facial preparation.

Here is a list of ingredients commonly used in facial preparations. By determining which of these ingredients contain the qualities you need, you can make up your own personalized facial pack.

MILK PRODUCTS contain natural skin-softeners and protein. In addition, sour milk and buttermilk are astringent.

> Buttermilk
> Cottage cheese
> Milk—skim, sour, powdered, or whole
> Sweet cream
> Yogurt

FRESH VEGETABLES contain astringents and natural vitamins which are absorbed by the skin. Among others:

> Artichokes   Cucumbers   Tomatoes
> Avocados   Potatoes

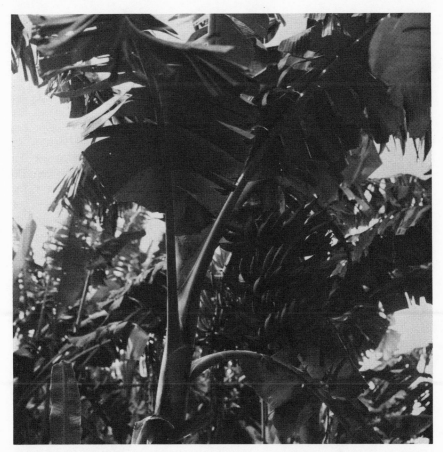

Bananas are used in facial preparations as an emollient. When the bunch is harvested, the plant is cut down. A new plant then grows from the roots. Arnold Krochmal.

FRESH FRUITS are astringent and contain vitamin C, some of which is absorbed through the skin. Citrus fruit peels contain natural oils which are beneficial to the skin.

Apples	Lemons	Papayas
· Bananas	Limes	Pineapples
Grapefruit	Oranges	Strawberries
Grapes		

NATURAL PLANT OILS are beneficial to the skin not only for their softening qualities, but for their vitamins as well.

Almond oil (as well as the meal)	Sunflower oil
Olive oil	Walnut oil
Strawberry oil	Wheat germ oil

Other sources of natural protein for the skin are eggs, gelatin, and brewers yeast. Honey is used in facials because it serves as a softener and binds the other ingredients together into a nice paste. Apple cider vinegar and wine vinegar are natural astringents. Oatmeal is soothing to the skin, and is higher in protein content than most grains.

Listed below are some of the herbs which are commonly used in facials.

Chamomile *Matricaria chamomilla*
Dandelion *Taraxacum officinale*
Elder flowers *Sambucus canadensis*
Hyssop *Hyssopus officinalis*
Lavender *Lavandula officinalis*
Linden flowers *Lindera benzoin*
Marigold *Calendula officinalis*

Mint *Mentha spicata*
Peppermint *Mentha piperita*
Rosemary *Rosmarinus officinalis*
Sage *Salvia officinalis*
Wild strawberry *Fragaria virginiana*
Yarrow *Achillea millefolium*

HERBAL FACIAL MASK

Oat flour or ground oatmeal	2 tablespoons
Arnica flowers	1 teaspoon
Chamomile flowers	1 teaspoon
Rosemary leaves	1/2 teaspoon
Water	2 tablespoons
Camphor	1/8 teaspoon

☛ Combine the flour and the herbs. Dissolve the camphor in the water, and add to the dry ingredients.

PROTEIN FACIAL MASK

Chick-pea flour	3 tablespoons
Rice flour	3 tablespoons
Tincture of benzoin	1 teaspoon
Rosewater	1 tablespoon
Honey	1 tablespoon
Beaten egg	1 small

☛ Combine the two flours, then add the other ingredients. Mix to a smooth paste.

BEAUTY CLAY

Kaolin	1/2 cup
Water	3/4 cup
Tincture of benzoin	1/2 teaspoon

☛ Combine the ingredients.

BEAUTY CLAY WITH GLYCERIN

Fuller's earth	1/2 cup
Glycerin	1 tablespoon
Water	1 tablespoon
Tincture of benzoin	2 tablespoons
Oil of bergamot	1/8 teaspoon

☛ Combine the ingredients.

FACE POWDER

The earliest face powders were wheat and rice flours, used by the ancient Jews, Assyrians, and Egyptians. Other natural untinted materials, such as lead powder, were used during the sixteenth and seventeenth centuries. All these were unsatisfactory because they were not the same color as the complexion and looked artificial and masklike. The rice powders irritated the skin by causing the pores to enlarge excessively. The lead powder was dangerous because it was absorbed through the skin into the blood system, and could eventually cause death.

The first tinted powder was made by Helena Rubinstein, using a talc base. Nowadays face powder is supplemented and used in conjunction with liquid and cream makeup, which contain powder in solution.

The average person would have a difficult time making up a satisfactory face powder because it is hard to achieve a suitable tint. Cosmetic chemists are able to do this because of the wide range of tints they have available.

ROUGES

The purpose of rouge is to simulate the rosy freshness of a young and healthy skin. It is one of the oldest types of makeup and is mentioned in Roman writings.

The modern rouge, or blusher, comes most commonly in a compact powder form, and is basically pressed powder with a large amount of color added. Rouges may also be obtained in liquid or cream form. The formulas I give are for a liquid or paste rouge.

LIQUID ROUGE [1]

Carmine	1/8 teaspoon
Ammonia	1/2 teaspoon
Alcohol	3 tablespoons
Oil of rose geranium	1/4 teaspoon
Rosewater	2 1/2 cups

☞ Mix the carmine with the ammonia, shaking until the carmine is thoroughly dissolved. Dissolve the oil in the alcohol, and add the rosewater. Combine with the ammonia mixture.

LIQUID ROUGE [2]

Carmine	1/8 teaspoon
Ammonia water	1 1/2 tablespoons
Alcohol	1 1/2 teaspoons
Oil of rose	5 drops

☞ Dissolve the carmine in the ammonia, and dissolve the oil in the alcohol. Combine the two mixtures. Let set 24 hours before using.

ROUGE [1]

Carmine	1/8 teaspoon
Talc	1 cup
Gum acacia	1 teaspoon
Ammonia	2 teaspoons

☞ Mix the carmine, talc, and gum acacia together in a blender. Transfer to a dish, and stir in a sufficient amount of ammonia, a few drops at a time, to make a stiff paste.

ROUGE [2]

Carmine	1/8 teaspoon
Talc	1 cup
Gum acacia	1 teaspoon
Water	2 teaspoons

☞ Grind the carmine, talc, and gum acacia together. Add enough water, a few drops at a time, to form a doughy mass.

ROUGE [3]

Carthamin	1/8 teaspoon
Talc	3/4 cup
Gum acacia	1 teaspoon
Oil of rose	5 drops

☞ Grind the carthamin, talc, and gum acacia together. Add the oil.

LIPSTICKS

Archaeologists have excavated lipsticks at the biblical city of Ur, and it is known that the Egyptians applied carmine color to their lips. The Greeks and Romans used a liquid or a paste, including carmine, to color their lips.

Lipstick in its present form is a relatively new item in cosmetics. Consisting of an all-wax base, with color, in the last thirty to forty years it has become a major money-maker for most cosmetic firms.

Lipstick is hard to make outside the laboratory. The exact shade of desired color must be achieved consistently by complete and thorough mixing; also the wax must be treated so it will not melt in the tube. The formulas included here are fairly simple, but they produce light-colored lip glosses rather than lipsticks.

COCOA BUTTER LIP GLOSS

Cocoa butter	4 tablespoons
Beeswax	1 teaspoon

☞ Melt the ingredients together over low heat.

COLD CREAM LIP GLOSS

Cold cream	1/2 cup
Glycerin	1 teaspoon
Tincture of benzoin	1/2 teaspoon
Carmine	1/8 teaspoon

☞ Mix the carmine with the glycerin. Add to the cold cream. Stir in the tincture of benzoin, and continue stirring until the alcohol has evaporated.

GLYCERIN LIP GLOSS

Cold cream	1/2 cup
Carmine	1/8 teaspoon
Glycerin	1 teaspoon

☞ Mix the carmine with the glycerin. Stir in the cold cream.

TINTED LIP GLOSS

Beeswax	2 tablespoons
Almond oil	1/4 cup
Carmine	1/8 teaspoon
Oil of rose	1 drop

☞ Melt the wax over low heat, and stir in the carmine. Gradually add the almond oil and the oil of rose.

LIQUID LIPSTICK [1]

Ammonia	1 tablespoon
Carmine	1 teaspoon

Alcohol	1 tablespoon
Oil of rose	5 drops
Rosewater	1 3/4 cups

☛ Combine the carmine and the ammonia, and let set for two days. Add the remaining ingredients, and let set again until the silt settles to the bottom. Pour the liquid into a container, and discard the silt.

LIQUID LIPSTICK [2]

Ammonia water	1/4 teaspoon
Carmine	1/8 teaspoon
Extract of rose	1/8 teaspoon
Rosewater	2 cups

☛ Soak the carmine in the ammonia water for two days. Add the remaining ingredients, and let set for a week, shaking frequently. Let set undisturbed until the liquid becomes clear.

EYE PREPARATIONS

Mascara, one of the most ancient of our cosmetics, has been used since biblical times. Eyeliners and shadows were first applied by the ancient Egyptians as a protection against excessive sun glare. The earliest known formula was commonly used by many peoples, including the East Indians, who mixed lampblack, or soot with oil. Football players still use this mixture today to minimize glare on the football field. Cleopatra, if current theater practice is historically accurate, carried eye makeup to an extreme.

Eyeliners, shadows, and mascara are difficult to prepare, to say the least, and the procedure requires elaborate equipment.

For the removal of eye makeup, the most gentle substance is mineral oil. The popular eye-makeup pads consist of mineral oil on a cotton applicator. Petroleum jelly may also be used.

ALMOND EYEBROW AND EYELASH SOFTENER

Castor oil	2 tablespoons
Almond oil	1/4 cup plus 2 tablespoons
Oil of rose	1 drop

☞ Combine the ingredients.

COCOA BUTTER EYEBROW AND EYELASH SOFTENER

Beeswax	1/2 cup
Cocoa butter	1/4 cup
Peanut oil	1/2 cup
Boric acid powder	1 teaspoon

☞ Melt the beeswax and the cocoa butter over low heat. Add the peanut oil and boric acid, stirring well.

EYEBROW AND EYELASH OIL

Castor oil	1 tablespoon plus 2 teaspoons
Walnut oil	5 tablespoons
Oil of rose	3 drops

☞ Combine the ingredients.

EYEBROW CREAM

Petroleum jelly	1/2 cup
Oil of lavender	5 drops
Oil of rosemary	5 drops

☞ Melt the petroleum jelly over low heat. Stir in the oils.

Hair Preparations

HAIR COLORINGS AND DYES

Hair dyes and colorings were used, according to records, by the ancient Egyptians, Greeks, Hebrews, Assyrians, Persians, Chinese, and Hindus. Henna is probably the oldest coloring perparation, followed by chamomile. The first recorded user of henna as a hair dye was the Egyptian queen, Ses, mother of King Teta in the Third Dynasty.

The desirable hair color at any given time is a quirk of fashion. When Queen Elizabeth came to the throne, blond hair was replaced by red hair because the Virgin Queen was a carrot-top. Only the people of the lower classes would still display blond hair.

All the formulas here call for natural vegetable materials, harmless to the hair and the skin. The color will wash out gradually with each shampoo. Even if the desired color is not achieved the first time, no permanent damage is done. The exact color produced by any preparation cannot be predicted, since each individual begins with a different shade of hair and the plant materials used are highly variable. A possible precaution would be to try the dye on a sample of hair that has been saved from a trim.

SHROPSHIRE HAIR COLORING (BLOND)

Rhubarb bark	1 cup
Alcohol	2 cups

☛ Soak the bark in the alcohol overnight, then strain.

VENETIAN HAIR COLORING (BLOND)

Honey	1/2 cup
Molasses	1/2 cup
Gum arabic	1 tablespoon

☛ Cook the ingredients in a double boiler for half an hour.

ELDER HAIR DYE (BLOND)

Elder bark	2 1/2 cups
Flowers of broom	3 cups
Egg yolk	1
Water	4 1/2 cups

☞ Boil all the ingredients together in a pot. Skim the oil from the top of the water as it appears. Continue cooking the mixture for about 30 minutes. Apply the oil to clean wet hair, leave it on the hair for 15 minutes, and then wash it out.

HENNA HAIR DYE (RED)

Henna leaves, crushed	2 tablespoons
Water	1 cup
Alcohol	1 tablespoon

☞ Crush the henna leaves and add to the warmed water. Let set overnight. Strain, and add the alcohol.

OLD ENGLISH HAIR DYE (RED)

Radish water	1 cup
Privet water	1 cup

☞ To make the radish water, combine 1/2 cup water with 1 cup sliced radishes in a blender. Blend to a puree, strain, and discard the solid material. To make the privet water, boil 1 cup of privet leaves with 1 1/2 cups of water for 30 minutes. Strain and add to the radish water.

INDIGO HAIR DYE (LIGHT BROWN)

Indigo	1/2 cup plus 1 tablespoon
Henna	1/4 cup
Water	1 cup

☞ Crush the indigo and the henna together. Add to the water and let set overnight. Strain.

ORANGE-FLOWER HAIR DYE (BROWN)

Gallnuts, crushed	2/3 cup
Water	1 cup plus 2 tablespoons
Orange-flower water	1 cup plus 2 tablespoons

☞ Boil the crushed gallnuts in the water for 15 minutes. Strain, and add the orange-flower water.

WALNUT HAIR DYE (BROWN)

Green walnut shells	3/4 cup
Alum	1/4 cup
Orange-flower water	3/4 cup

☞ Grind the walnut shells to a powder. Add the alum, and moisten with the orange-flower water.

INDIGO HAIR DYE (BLACK)

Indigo	1/4 cup
Henna	1/2 teaspoon
Water	1/2 cup

☞ Grind the indigo and the henna together. Add to the water, and let set overnight. Strain.

INDIAN HAIR DYE (BLACK)

Gum arabic	2 teaspoons
India ink	2 tablespoons
Orange-flower water	3 cups

☞ Add the gum arabic and the india ink to the orange-flower water, and let set overnight.

WALNUT HAIR DYE (BLACK)

Walnut shells, green	1/2 cup
Alum	2 teaspoons
Peanut oil	2 cups

☞ Grind the walnut shells with the alum. Add to the peanut oil, and stir over low heat until any moisture evaporates.

DYE FOR GRAY HAIR (RESTORES NATURAL COLOR)

Peanut oil	1 cup
Orange peel, dried and sliced	1/2 cup
Alcohol	1/2 cup

☞ Add the alcohol to the orange peel, and let set in a bottle for four days. Strain, and discard the peel. Add the alcohol mixture to the peanut oil, and let set for two weeks before using.

HAIR CONDITIONERS, DRESSINGS, AND TONICS

The Egyptians and Romans were among the first to use hair dressings. Their elaborate hair styles required generous amounts of dressings and pomades. For long ceremonies, tiny wax balls, heavily perfumed, were worn within the headdress; as these melted in warm air, they would perfume and oil the hair. Roman pomades had animal fat as a base. An apple was pierced with cloves, cinnamon, and other spices and placed in the rendered fat, which picked up the smell of the spices. The perfumed fat was then applied to the hair.

A hair tonic, when massaged into the scalp and hair, stimulates the flow of oils and of blood in the scalp, and may also be antiseptic. A hair tonic consists largely of alcohol in which some oil, such as mineral or castor oil, is dissolved, plus scent.

Hair conditioners and dressings are used mainly to help style the hair according to particular ideas of taste and grooming. In addition, they also condition dry hair by adding oils.

ALMOND HAIR CONDITIONER

Almond oil	2 tablespoons
Tincture of benzoin	1 teaspoon
Alcohol	3/4 cup

☞ Dissolve the almond oil in the alcohol, and then add the tincture of benzoin. Massage this preparation into the scalp daily to promote blood circulation.

BARBERRY HAIR CONDITIONER

Barberry bark	3 cups
Water	4 cups

☞ Boil the bark until half of the water evaporates. Rinse the hair twice a day in this liquid.

BAY HAIR CONDITIONER

Borax	1 teaspoon
Glycerin	1 1/2 teaspoons
Potassium carbonate	1/2 teaspoon
Alcohol	2 tablespoons
Oil of bay	1/4 teaspoon
Water	1 cup

☞ Dissolve the borax and potassium carbonate in the water. Dissolve the oil in the alcohol. Combine the mixtures, and add the glycerin.

NETTLE HAIR CONDITIONER

Expressed juice of fresh nettle	1 cup

☞ Comb this into the hair in the morning.

SOUTHERNWOOD HAIR CONDITIONER

Southernwood herb	4 cups
Vegetable oil	1 1/2 cups
Burgundy wine	1/2 cup

☞ Bring all the ingredients to a boil, and simmer for half an hour. Drain.

BERGAMOT HAIR DRESSING

Quince seed	1 tablespoon
Water, hot	1 cup
Alcohol	1 cup
Oil of bergamot	1/2 teaspoon

☞ Combine the water and quince seeds. Let set to form a mucilage. Dissolve the oil of bergamot in the alcohol. Strain the mucilage, and add the alcohol.

COCOA BUTTER HAIR DRESSING

Cocoa butter	1 tablespoon
Almond oil	1 cup
Glycerin	1 1/2 tablespoons
Alcohol	2 tablespoons

☞ Melt the cocoa butter over low heat. Stir in the almond oil and glycerin. Add the alcohol.

COCONUT OIL HAIR DRESSING

Coconut oil	2 tablespoons
Walnut oil	1 cup
Alcohol	3/4 cup plus 2 tablespoons
Oil of bergamot	1/4 teaspoon
Oil of cinnamon	1/8 teaspoon

☞ Liquefy the coconut oil over low heat. Dissolve the walnut oil and the oils of bergamot and cinnamon in the alcohol, and add to the coconut oil.

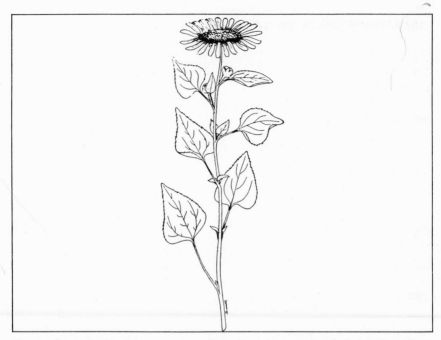

The sunflower is found in a great number of species, ranging in height from three feet to twelve feet or more. Sunflower-seed oil is used in creams of all sorts, and the dried flowers are used in facial packs, herbal baths, and as a hair dye. (Helianthus spp.) University of Colorado.

ROSEMARY HAIR DRESSING

Coconut oil	1 cup
Mineral oil	3/4 cup
Alcohol	1/4 cup
Oil of rosemary	1/4 teaspoon
Oil of lemon	1/8 teaspoon

☞ Liquefy the coconut oil over low heat and add the mineral oil. Dissolve the oils of rosemary and lemon in the alcohol, and add to the coconut oil.

SUNFLOWER HAIR DRESSING

Lanolin	3 tablespoons
Sunflower oil	1/2 cup
Soap flakes	1 teaspoon
Water, hot	1 1/4 cups
Rosewater	1/4 cup

☞ Melt the lanolin over low heat. Add the sunflower oil. Dissolve the soap in the water, and add the rosewater. Combine the two mixtures.

ASTRINGENT HAIR TONIC

Alcohol	1 cup
Castor oil	1 tablespoon
Mineral oil	1 tablespoon

☞ Combine the ingredients.

BAY RUM HAIR TONIC

Alcohol	1 2/3 cups
Water	1 2/3 cups
New England rum	3/4 cup
Oil of bay	1 teaspoon
Oil of pimento	1/4 teaspoon

☞ Dissolve the oils in the alcohol. Add the rum and the water.

CHAMOMILE HAIR TONIC

Sage	1/2 cup
Chamomile flowers	1/4 cup
Alcohol	1 1/2 cups
Mineral oil	3 tablespoons

☞ Let the sage and chamomile steep in the alcohol for 24 hours. Strain, and add the mineral oil.

LEMON HAIR TONIC

Alcohol	1 1/2 cups
Water	3/4 cup
Menthol	1 teaspoon
Oil of lemon	1/2 teaspoon

☞ Dissolve the menthol and oil in the alcohol. Add the water.

NETTLE HAIR TONIC

Rosemary	1/4 cup
Nettle	1/2 cup

Almond oil	2 tablespoons
Alcohol	2 cups

☞ Let the rosemary and nettle steep in the alcohol for two days. Strain, and add the almond oil.

ROSE HAIR TONIC

Alcohol	3 tablespoons
Oil of rosemary	1/8 teaspoon
Oil of cinnamon	1/8 teaspoon
Rosewater	1/4 cup plus 1 tablespoon

☞ Dissolve the oils in the alcohol. Add the rosewater.

ROSEMARY HAIR TONIC

Water	1 cup
Alcohol	1 cup
Rosemary	1/2 cup
Sage	1/2 cup
Boric acid powder	1/2 teaspoon

☞ Let the rosemary and sage steep in the alcohol for 24 hours. Strain, and add the boric acid powder and water.

SAGE HAIR TONIC

Tincture of green soap	1 cup
Glycerin	1 tablespoon
Menthol	2 teaspoons
Oil of bay	1/4 teaspoon
Oil of sage	1/8 teaspoon
Alcohol	1 cup
Water	3/4 cup

☞ Dissolve the menthol and the oils in the alcohol. Add the water and glycerin. Gently stir in the tincture of green soap.

STRAWBERRY HERB HAIR TONIC

Rosemary	1/4 cup
Strawberry herb	1/4 cup
Sage	2 tablespoons
Mineral oil	1/4 cup
Alcohol	1 cup and 2 tablespoons
Water	1/4 cup

☞ Let the rosemary, strawberry herb, and sage steep in the alcohol for two days. Strain, then add the mineral oil and the water.

SOME PLANTS USED TO TREAT HAIR

Name	Part Used	Botanical Name
Apache plume	Leaves	*Fallugia*
Leatherstem	Foliage	*Jatropia*
Maidenhair fern	Foliage	*Adiantum*
Weld gourd	Seeds	*Cucurbita*
Yucca	Foliage	*Yucca*

HAIR WASHES AND RINSES

Hair washes and rinses are used to remove soap scum left in the hair after shampooing; to leave the hair smooth and manageable; and to restore the natural oils lost in shampooing. Vinegar and lemon juice are common rinses and have been used for centuries. Many rinses include herbs, such as rosemary, whose virtues have been thought to be almost magical. Most of the formulas I give here are very, very old, including some from Greece and Rome, and some from Europe that are at least five hundred years old.

BAY RUM HAIR WASH

Ammonium carbonate	1 1/2 tablespoons
Borax	1 1/2 tablespoons
Orange-flower water	1 1/4 cups
Alcohol	1/2 cup
Oil of bay	1/8 teaspoon
Oil of rosemary	5 drops

☞ Dissolve the oils in the alcohol. Combine the ammonium carbonate, borax, and orange-flower water. Add to the alcohol mixture.

DELPHIC HAIR WASH

Rosewater	1 cup
Orange-flower water	1 cup
Alcohol	1/4 cup
Sassafras wood chips	1 cup
Potassium carbonate	1 teaspoon

☞ Soak the sassafras chips in the alcohol for three days. Strain, then add the rosewater. Dissolve the potassium carbonate in the orange-flower water, and add to the first mixture.

FLORAL HAIR WASH

Liquid soap	1/2 teaspoon
Rosewater	1 1/2 cups
Glycerin	3 tablespoons
Alcohol	3 tablespoons
Oil of orange	1/4 teaspoon
Ammonia	1 teaspoon

☞ Dissolve the oil of orange in the alcohol. Add the rosewater and glycerin. Stir in the soap, and add the ammonia.

LAUREL HAIR WASH

Ammonium carbonate	1 tablespoon
Borax	1/2 cup
Orange-flower water	1 1/2 cups
Alcohol	3/4 cup
Oil of laurel	1/4 teaspoon
Oil of orange	1/4 teaspoon

☞ Dissolve the ammonium carbonate and the borax in the orange-flower water. Dissolve the oils in the alcohol, and combine the mixtures.

ROSE HAIR WASH

Potassium carbonate	2 teaspoons
Rosemary water	1 cup
Rosewater	1/2 cup
Alcohol	1/2 cup plus 2 tablespoons
Oil of rose	5 drops

☞ Dissolve the potassium carbonate in the rosewater, and add the rosemary water. Dissolve the oil of rose in the alcohol, and combine with the first mixture.

ROSEMARY HAIR WASH

Alcohol	1/4 cup
Rosemary water	3 cups
Boric acid powder	1 teaspoon

☞ Dissolve the boric acid in the rosemary water. Add the alcohol.

SOAP HAIR WASH

Glycerin	1/4 cup
Alcohol	1 cup
Water, hot	3/4 cup
Soap flakes	2 teaspoons
Oil of patchouly	1/8 teaspoon

☞ Dissolve the oil in the alcohol. Dissolve the soap in the water, and add the glycerin. Combine the two mixtures.

HERBAL AFTER-SHAMPOO RINSE

Sage	1/2 cup
Rosemary	1/2 cup
Sassafras wood chips	1/4 cup
Water	3 cups
Boric acid powder	1 teaspoon

☞ Heat the water to boiling, and combine with the sage, rosemary, and the sassafras chips. Let the mixture set for 12 hours, then strain. Add the boric acid.

AFTER-SHAMPOO RINSE

Lemon juice, fresh; or white vinegar	1 cup
Water	1 cup

☞ Mix this at time of use.

SHAMPOOS

Shampoos are used to remove foreign matter, loose skin, dirt, and excess oils from the scalp and hair. They should clean well but should not strip the hair of its natural oils. Shampoos come in various forms— liquid, cream, paste, and powder. The basic ingredients are alcohol, glycerin, soap, scents, tints, water, and sometimes protein in the form of egg, gelatin, and casein.

BALSAM SHAMPOO

Soap flakes	2 tablespoons
Potassium carbonate	3 1/2 tablespoons
Water, hot	1 1/2 cups
Alcohol	1/4 cup
Oil of balsam	1/4 teaspoon

☞ Dissolve the soap and potassium carbonate in the water. Dissolve the oil of balsam in the alcohol. Combine the two mixtures.

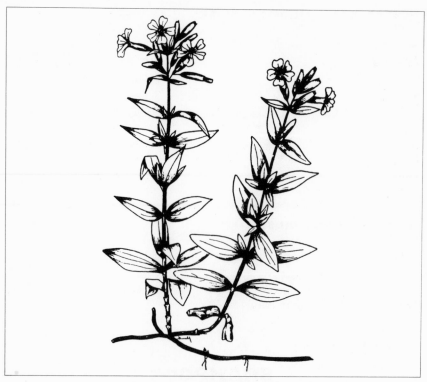

Bouncing bet, or soapwort, is a weed found all over the United States. Growing to three feet in height, it has been used as a soap substitute and for shampoos. (Saponaria spp.) University of Colorado.

BAY SHAMPOO

Soap flakes	3 tablespoons
Potassium carbonate	1 1/2 tablespoons
Water, hot	1 cup
Oil of bay	1/4 teaspoon
Alcohol	2 tablespoons

Dissolve the soap and potassium carbonate in the water. Dissolve the oil of bay in the alcohol, and add to the first mixture.

BAY RUM SHAMPOO

Soap flakes	2 tablespoons
Ammonia water	2 tablespoons
Water, hot	1 cup

| Alcohol | 2 tablespoons |
| Oil of bay | 1/4 teaspoon |

☞ Dissolve the soap in the water. Dissolve the oil of bay in the alcohol, and add to the water-soap mixture. Stir in the ammonia water.

MARTINIQUE BAY RUM SHAMPOO

Borax	4 tablespoons
Glycerin	3 tablespoons
Egg whites	2
Alcohol	1 cup
Water	1 1/2 cups
Oil of bay	1/4 teaspoon

☞ Dissolve the oil in the alcohol, and the borax in the water. Beat the egg whites to a froth. Combine the water mixture with the alcohol and egg whites. Stir in the glycerin.

BERGAMOT SHAMPOO

Ammonia	1 tablespoon plus 2 teaspoons
Glycerin	3 tablespoons
Soap flakes	1/2 cup
Alcohol	3/4 cup
Water, hot	3 cups
Oil of bergamot	1 teaspoon

☞ Dissolve the oil in the alcohol, and add the glycerin. Dissolve the soap in the water, and add to the first mixture. Stir in the ammonia.

LEMON-EGG SHAMPOO

Egg yolks	2
Soap flakes	1 tablespoon
Ammonia water	1 tablespoon
Alcohol	1 teaspoon
Oil of lemon	1/4 teaspoon
Water, hot	1 3/4 cups

☞ Dissolve the oil in the alcohol. Dissolve the soap in the water, and add the beaten egg yolks. Combine the alcohol and the water mixture. Stir in the ammonia water.

ONE-EGG SHAMPOO

Egg, whole	1
Soap flakes	2 tablespoons
Water, hot	1 cup
Alcohol	1 teaspoon
Potassium carbonate	1 teaspoon
Oil of sweet almond	1 teaspoon
Ammonia water	1/4 teaspoon

☞ Dissolve the soap and potassium carbonate in the water. Dissolve the oil in the alcohol, and add to the water mixture. Beat the egg well, and add to the first mixture. Stir in the ammonia water.

RICH EGG SHAMPOO

Egg white	1
Water	1/2 cup plus 2 tablespoons
Cologne water	2 tablespoons
Alcohol	1/2 cup

☞ Beat the egg white to a froth. Combine the other ingredients and add to the egg white.

EVERGLADES SHAMPOO

Soap flakes	1/4 cup
Potassium carbonate	1 1/2 tablespoons
Alcohol	1 cup
Water, hot	2 cups
Oil of lime	1/4 teaspoon

☞ Dissolve the soap and potassium carbonate in the water. Dissolve the oil in the alcohol, and add to the water mixture.

FLORENTINE SHAMPOO

Borax	2 tablespoons
Potassium carbonate	1 tablespoon
Water, hot	2 cups
Alcohol	2 cups

Oil of lemon	1/4 teaspoon
Oil of rosemary	1/8 teaspoon
Ammonia water	2 teaspoons

☛ Dissolve the borax and potassium carbonate in the water. Dissolve the oils in the alcohol, and add to the water mixture. Stir in the ammonia water.

GLYCERIN SHAMPOO

Soap flakes	2 cups
Water, hot	1 1/2 cups
Glycerin	1/2 cup
Oil of orange	1/4 teaspoon
Oil of patchouly	1/4 teaspoon
Alcohol	1 tablespoon

☛ Dissolve the soap in the water. Dissolve the oils in the alcohol, and add to the water mixture. Stir in the glycerin.

JASMINE SHAMPOO

Soap flakes	1/4 cup
Potassium carbonate	1 tablespoon
Oil of jasmine	1/4 teaspoon
Alcohol	1/2 cup
Water, hot	2 cups

☛ Dissolve the soap and potassium carbonate in the water. Dissolve the oil in the alcohol, and add to the water mixture.

LAVENDER SHAMPOO

Ammonium carbonate	1 tablespoon
Borax	1 tablespoon
Tincture of benzoin	1 1/2 teaspoons
Glycerin	1 1/2 teaspoons
Alcohol	1 cup
Water	1 cup
Lavender water	1/3 cup

☛ Dissolve the ammonium carbonate and borax in the water. Add the remaining ingredients.

LEMON SHAMPOO

Soap flakes	1/3 cup
Potassium carbonate	2 tablespoons
Water, hot	2 cups
Oil of lemon	1/4 teaspoon
Alcohol	1/2 cup

☞ Dissolve the soap and potassium carbonate in the water. Dissolve the oil in the alcohol, and add to the water mixture.

SAN FERNANDO VALLEY LEMON SHAMPOO

Potassium carbonate	1 tablespoon
Ammonium carbonate	2 tablespoons
Soap flakes	2 tablespoons
Borax	1 tablespoon
Water, hot	1 3/4 cups
Alcohol	3 tablespoons
Oil of lemon	1 teaspoon

☞ Dissolve the first four ingredients in the water. Dissolve the oil in the alcohol, and add to the water mixture.

LEMON GRASS SHAMPOO

Potassium carbonate	2 tablespoons
Ammonium carbonate	1 tablespoon
Soap flakes	1/4 cup
Water, hot	1 3/4 cups
Alcohol	3 tablespoons
Oil of lemon grass	1/4 teaspoon

☞ Dissolve the first three ingredients in the water. Dissolve the oil in the alcohol, and add to the water mixture.

MEDICATED SHAMPOO

Menthol	1/4 teaspoon
Oil of eucalyptus	1/8 teaspoon
Alcohol	2 tablespoons

| Soap flakes | 2 tablespoons |
| Water, hot | 1/4 cup |

☛ Dissolve the menthol and oil in the alcohol. Dissolve the soap in the water, and add to the alcohol mixture.

NEROLI SHAMPOO

Potassium carbonate	2 tablespoons
Water, hot	2 cups
Ammonia water	1 tablespoon
Mineral oil	1 tablespoon
Oil of neroli	1/4 teaspoon

☛ Dissolve the potassium carbonate in the water. Add the oils, mix, and add the ammonia water.

JAFFA ORANGE SHAMPOO

Tincture of green soap	1/4 cup
Potassium carbonate	1 1/2 teaspoons
Water, hot	1 3/4 cups
Oil of jaffa orange	1/4 teaspoon

☛ Dissolve the potassium carbonate in the water. Combine the oil and the tincture of green soap and combine with the water mixture.

ORANGE SHAMPOO

Ammonium carbonate	1 tablespoon
Borax	1 1/2 tablespoons
Glycerin	2 tablespoons
Orange-flower water	1 1/2 cups
Oil of orange	1/8 teaspoon
Alcohol	2 cups

☛ Dissolve the ammonium carbonate and borax in the orange-flower water. Add the glycerin. Dissolve the oil in the alcohol, and combine with the first mixture.

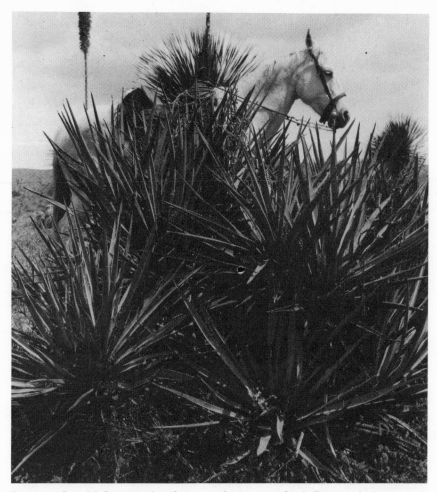

Yucca, or Spanish bayonet, has been used as a soap by Indians and pioneers. It is found in the warmer parts of the United States. (Yucca spp.) U.S. Forest Service.

GEORGIA PINES SHAMPOO

Soap flakes	1 tablespoon
Potassium carbonate	1 teaspoon
Borax	1 teaspoon
Water, hot	1 cup
Alcohol	1 tablespoon
Oil of pine	1/8 teaspoon

☞ Dissolve the first three ingredients in the water. Dissolve the oil in the alcohol, and add to the water mixture.

PROTEIN SHAMPOO

Egg white	1
Glycerin	1 tablespoon
Oil of bay	1/8 teaspoon
Water	1/2 cup plus 2 tablespoons
Alcohol	1/2 cup
Borax	3 tablespoons

☞ Beat the egg white to a froth, and add the glycerin. Combine the borax and water, and add to the egg mixture. Dissolve the oil in the alcohol, and add to the first mixture.

ROSE SHAMPOO

Potassium carbonate	2 tablespoons
Borax	2 tablespoons
Water, hot	1 cup
Rosewater	1 cup

☞ Dissolve the potassium carbonate and borax in the water. Add the rosewater.

SHAMPOO FOR OILY HAIR

Soap flakes	2 tablespoons
Water, hot	1/4 cup
Alcohol	1 cup

☞ Dissolve the soap in the water. Add the alcohol.

OIL SHAMPOO

Castor oil	1/4 cup
Water	1/4 cup

☞ Heat the water to lukewarm, and add the oil. This must be freshly prepared at the time of use.

PEANUT OIL SHAMPOO

Alcohol	2 tablespoons
Peanut oil	1/2 cup
Castor oil	1/4 cup
Water	3/4 cup

☞ Heat the water to lukewarm, and add the alcohol. Stir in the oils.

SUNFLOWER OIL SHAMPOO

Sunflower oil	1/4 cup
Almond oil	1/4 cup
Tincture of green soap	1 cup

☞ Combine the ingredients.

TIBETAN OIL SHAMPOO

Sesame oil	1 teaspoon
Mineral oil	1 teaspoon
Alcohol	1 cup
Water, warm	2 cups
Ammonium carbonate	1 tablespoon
Ammonia water	1 1/2 teaspoons

☞ Dissolve the ammonium carbonate in the water. Dissolve the sesame and mineral oils in the alcohol. Add to the water mixture. Stir in the ammonia water.

BERGAMOT SHAMPOO CONCENTRATE

Soap flakes	1/4 cup
Potassium carbonate	3/4 cup
Glycerin	1 cup
Water, hot	1 cup
Oil of rosemary	1/4 teaspoon
Oil of bergamot	1/4 teaspoon

☞ Dissolve the potassium carbonate and soap in the water. Add the glycerin and the oils.

LEMON SHAMPOO CONCENTRATE

Potassium carbonate	1/4 cup
Glycerin	1/4 cup
Water, hot	3 tablespoons
Soap flakes	1/4 cup
Alcohol	1/4 cup
Oil of lemon	1/2 teaspoon

☞ Dissolve the potassium carbonate and soap in the water, and add the glycerin. Dissolve the oil in the alcohol and add to the first mixture.

BLUEBERRY SHAMPOO POWDER*

Soap flakes	1/2 cup
Borax	3/4 cup
Oil of cinnamon	5 drops
Oil of blueberry	1/4 teaspoon

☞ Combine the soap and borax. Stir in the oils.

CHAMOMILE SHAMPOO POWDER

Soap flakes	1/2 cup
Borax	1 1/2 teaspoons
Baking soda	1 teaspoon
Potassium carbonate	1 teaspoon
Chamomile flowers, ground	2 tablespoons

☞ Combine the ingredients.

HERBAL SHAMPOO POWDER

Ammonium carbonate	1/4 cup
Borax	1/4 cup
Sage, ground	1/4 cup
Oil of sage	1/8 teaspoon

☞ Combine the ammonium carbonate, borax, and sage. Stir in the oil.

* When using a shampoo powder, dissolve 2 tablespoons of the powder in 1/4 cup of warm water.

LAVENDER SHAMPOO POWDER

Potassium carbonate	3 tablespoons
Borax	3 tablespoons
Soap flakes	2 tablespoons
Oil of lavender	1/4 teaspoon

☞ Combine the potassium carbonate, borax, and soap. Stir in the oil.

LINDEN FLOWERS SHAMPOO POWDER

Potassium carbonate	3 tablespoons
Soap flakes	1/4 cup
Borax	3 tablespoons
Linden flowers, ground	2 tablespoons

☞ Combine the ingredients.

ORANGE SHAMPOO POWDER

Soap flakes	1 cup
Borax	1 cup
Baking soda	1 tablespoon
Ground orange peel	1 teaspoon
Oil of orange	1/4 teaspoon

☞ Combine the soap, borax, baking soda, and orange peel. Stir in the oil.

ROSE SHAMPOO POWDER

Cornstarch	2 tablespoons
Fuller's earth	1 cup
Soap flakes	1/4 cup
Orrisroot powder	1/3 cup
Alcohol	2 tablespoons
Rose petals, crushed	1/4 cup

☞ Mix the ingredients well.

STRAWBERRY SHAMPOO POWDER

Borax	3/4 cup
Sodium carbonate	1/2 cup
Soap flakes	1/2 cup
Oil of strawberry	1/4 teaspoon

☞ Combine the borax, sodium carbonate, and soap. Add the oil.

DRY SHAMPOO (to be used without water)

Rice flour	1/2 cup
Baking soda	1 teaspoon
Borax	1 1/2 tablespoons

☞ Mix well. Massage into the hair and scalp with the fingers. Use a hairbrush to remove the excess powder. This is for use mainly when you are in a hurry and haven't time for the usual shampoo.

WAVESETS AND HAIR-SETTING LOTIONS

Wavesets were first made by the pharaohic Egyptians, with some of the same seeds and gums as are used now. A modern waveset or setting lotion consists of plant gum or seeds soaked in water or some other liquid to form a mucilage; perfume; coloring matter; and usually a high percentage of alcohol. The mucilage surrounds the hair and helps it to curl in the desired fashion. As time goes by, the mucilage will start to disappear from the hair and the hair will begin to lose its curl.

ELDER-FLOWER HAIR-CURLING WASH

Gum arabic	2 teaspoons
Powdered sugar	1 teaspoon
Elder-flower water	1/2 cup

☞ Soften the gum in the elder-flower water. Add the sugar.

LAVENDER HAIR-CURLING WASH

Tragacanth	1 tablespoon
Lavender water	1 cup
Water, hot	1 cup

☛ Combine the water and tragacanth, and let set to form a mucilage. Add the lavender water.

ORANGE-FLOWER HAIR-CURLING WASH

Gum arabic	1 tablespoon
Boric acid powder	1 1/2 tablespoons
Water, hot	1 cup
Orange-flower water	3/4 cup
Sugar	2 tablespoons

☛ Combine the water and gum, stirring until the mixture is smooth. Mix in the boric acid and the sugar and add the orange-flower water.

TRAGACANTH HAIR-CURLING WASH

Tragacanth	1 1/2 teaspoons
Glycerin	1 tablespoon
Alcohol	1 teaspoon
Water, hot	1/2 cup

☛ Mix the tragacanth with the glycerin. Add the water, and alcohol.

BENZOIN WAVING LOTION [1]

Tincture of benzoin	3 tablespoons
Alcohol	3/4 cup plus 2 tablespoons
Oil of lemon	1/4 teaspoon

☛ Dissolve the oil in the alcohol. Add to the tincture of benzoin.

BENZOIN WAVING LOTION [2]

Water	1 1/2 cups
Glycerin	1 tablespoon
Borax	1 1/2 tablespoons
Tincture of benzoin	1/2 cup

☛ Dissolve the borax in the water. Add the glycerin and the tincture of benzoin.

GLYCERIN WAVING LOTION

Gum karaya	1 teaspoon
Glycerin	1 teaspoon
Alcohol	1 1/2 tablespoons
Boric acid powder	1/2 teaspoon
Water	1/2 cup

☛ Stir the gum into the glycerin until it softens. Add the water gradually, then add the alcohol and the boric acid.

LEMON WAVING LOTION

Gum karaya	2 tablespoons
Glycerin	1 tablespoon
Alcohol	2 tablespoons
Oil of lemon	1/4 teaspoon
Water	2 cups

☛ Stir the gum in the glycerin until it softens. Dissolve the oil in the alcohol. Combine the two mixtures and add the water.

ORANGE-FLOWER WAVING LOTION

Potassium carbonate	1 tablespoon
Glycerin	1 tablespoon
Alcohol	1 tablespoon
Orange-flower water	1 cup
Water	1 cup
Ammonia	1/4 teaspoon

☛ Dissolve the potassium carbonate in the water. Add the remaining ingredients.

PSYLLIUM-SEED WAVING LOTION

Psyllium seed	1 tablespoon
Water, hot	2 cups
Alcohol	1/2 cup

☞ Combine the psyllium seed and water, and let set for 15 minutes to form a mucilage. Strain, and add the alcohol.

QUINCE-SEED WAVING LOTION

Quince seed	2 teaspoons
Alcohol	1/2 cup
Water, hot	1/2 cup

☞ Combine the quince seed and water, and let set to form a mucilage. Add the alcohol.

ROSE WAVING LOTION

Potassium carbonate	1 tablespoon
Glycerin	1 tablespoon
Water	1 cup
Rosewater	1 cup
Ammonia	1/2 teaspoon

☞ Dissolve the potassium carbonate in the water. Add the remaining ingredients.

ROSE-GLYCERIN WAVING LOTION

Potassium carbonate	2 teaspoons
Glycerin	2 teaspoons
Alcohol	3 tablespoons
Rosewater	1 cup
Water	1 cup

☞ Dissolve the potassium carbonate in the water. Add the remaining ingredients.

TRAGACANTH WAVING LOTION [1]

Tragacanth	1 tablespoon
Alcohol	1/4 cup
Water	1 3/4 cups
Borax	1/2 teaspoon
Boric acid powder	1/2 teaspoon

☞ Soak the tragacanth in the water until it softens. Dissolve the borax and boric acid in the alcohol, and add to the first mixture.

TRAGACANTH WAVING LOTION [2]

Tragacanth	2 teaspoons
Alcohol	1/4 cup plus 2 tablespoons
Rosewater	1/4 cup
Water	1/2 cup
Potassium carbonate	1 1/2 teaspoons
Borax	3 tablespoons

☞ Soak the tragacanth in the water until it softens. Add the potassium carbonate and the borax, and stir until dissolved. Stir in the alcohol and rosewater.

TRAGACANTH WAVING LOTION [3]

Tragacanth	2 teaspoons
Potassium carbonate	2 tablespoons
Boric acid powder	1 tablespoon
Alcohol	1/3 cup
Water	1 3/4 cups
Oil of lemon	1/4 teaspoon

☞ Soak the tragacanth in the water until it softens. Add the potassium carbonate and the boric acid. Dissolve the oil in the alcohol, and add to the first mixture.

WAVING LOTION

Gum acacia	1 1/2 teaspoons
Boric acid powder	1 teaspoon
Alcohol	3 tablespoons
Water	2 cups

☛ Mix the gum with a small amount of the water until it is dissolved. Dissolve the boric acid in the rest of the water, and add to the gum mixture. Stir in the alcohol.

Lotions, Creams, Conditioners

Lotions and creams usually consist of emollients or softeners, scent, water, and alcohol. The emollients, such as lanolin and glycerin, soothe and soften the skin, and replace some of the natural moisture lost by the skin. Many emollients are also found in plants, and I have included several. Usually in the form of a wax or fat, the emollient also acts as an agent to hold the water on the skin long enough for it to be absorbed, rather than evaporating immediately.

While lotions are related to cold creams, they are used for moisturizing rather than cleansing. During the day, women often prefer to use a lotion or greaseless cream under their makeup.

There are many types of lotions and creams, with or without alcohol. The most famous of these is rosewater and glycerin, which may be either a lotion or a cream.

LOTIONS

ALMOND LOTION

Almonds, sliced	1/2 cup
Soap flakes	1 tablespoon
Oil of bitter almond	5 drops
Oil of bergamot	10 drops
Alcohol	1/2 cup
Rosewater	1 1/2 cups

☞ Dissolve the oils in the alcohol. Combine the rosewater and almonds in a blender, and add the alcohol mixture. Stir in the soap.

CUCUMBER LOTION

Cucumber, large	1
Water, hot	1 cup
Boric acid powder	1/4 teaspoon
Glycerin	1/4 cup
Tincture of benzoin	1 teaspoon

☞ Pour the water over the sliced, unpeeled cucumbers. When the cucumbers become pulpy, squeeze through muslin to remove the juice. Combine the juice with the remaining ingredients.

FLORAL LOTION

Glycerin	1/2 cup
Alcohol	3 tablespoons
Oil of neroli	8 drops
Oil of bergamot	10 drops
Oil of jasmine	7 drops
Oil of lemon	1/8 teaspoon
Water	1 1/4 cups
Borax	1 1/2 teaspoons
Orange-flower water	1/4 cup

☞ Dissolve the oils in the alcohol. Add the glycerin and the orange-flower water. Dissolve the borax in the water, and add to the first mixture.

FLORAL GLYCERIN LOTION

Glycerin	1/4 cup plus 2 tablespoons
Rosewater or orange-flower water	1 cup

☞ Combine and shake well.

LANOLIN LOTION

Lanolin	2 tablespoons
Borax	1/4 teaspoon
Soap flakes	1/4 teaspoon
Water, hot	1/3 cup

☞ Dissolve the soap and lanolin in the water. Add the borax.

LEMON JUICE LOTION

Pectin	1/4 teaspoon
Lemon juice	2 teaspoons
Water, hot	1/2 cup
Glycerin	1/4 cup
Boric acid powder	1/2 teaspoon

☞ Dissolve the boric acid and pectin in the water. Add the lemon juice and glycerin.

MINT LOTION

Tragacanth	1 teaspoon
Water, hot	1/3 cup
Alcohol	1/2 cup
Glycerin	2 tablespoons
Menthol	1/4 teaspoon
Oil of peppermint	1/4 teaspoon

☞ Soak the tragacanth in the water to form a mucilage. Dissolve the oil of peppermint and menthol in the alcohol, and add the glycerin. Combine the mucilage with the alcohol mixture.

QUINCE-SEED LOTION

Quince seeds	1 teaspoon
Soap flakes	1/4 teaspoon
Boric acid powder	1/4 teaspoon
Alcohol	1 teaspoon
Glycerin	2 tablespoons
Water, hot	1 cup

☞ Soak the quince seeds in the water to form a mucilage. Strain, then add the remaining ingredients.

SMOOTH ROSE LOTION

Tincture of benzoin	1 tablespoon
Rosewater	1 cup
Glycerin	2 tablespoons

☞ Combine the ingredients.

ROSE LOTION

Tincture of benzoin	1 tablespoon
Rosewater	1 cup

☞ Combine the ingredients.

SOFT LOTION

Tragacanth	1 teaspoon
Water, hot	1 cup
Boric acid powder	1/4 teaspoon
Glycerin	1 tablespoon
Alcohol	1 tablespoon

☞ Soak the tragacanth in the water to form a mucilage. Dissolve the boric acid in the alcohol, and add the glycerin. Combine the two mixtures.

WITCH HAZEL LOTION

Alcohol	1/4 cup plus 2 tablespoons
Menthol	1/8 teaspoon
Baking soda	1 tablespoon
Witch hazel	1/4 cup plus 2 tablespoons
Water	1 1/4 cups

☞ Dissolve the menthol in the alcohol. Add the baking soda and the witch hazel. Add the water and stir briskly. (This lotion is not recommended for delicate skins.)

ROSE–WITCH HAZEL LOTION

Glycerin	1/2 cup
Rosewater	1/4 cup
Witch hazel	1/4 cup

☞ Combine the ingredients.

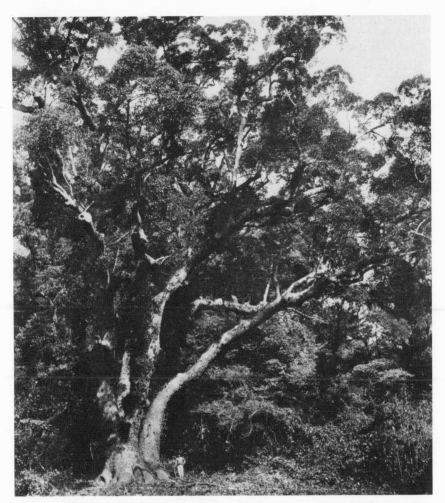

A 300-year-old camphor tree in Japan. **Camphor is used cosmetically as a pre-servative and fixative in colognes.** (Cinnamomum camphora) U.S. Forest Service.

ALMOND HAND LOTION

Alcohol	1/2 cup
Camphor	2 teaspoons
Glycerin	2 tablespoons
Water	1 cup
Oil of sweet almond	1/2 teaspoon

☞ Dissolve the camphor and the oil in the alcohol. Add the water and glycerin.

HAND LOTION

Boric acid powder	1 teaspoon
Glycerin	2 1/2 tablespoons
Lanolin	3 tablespoons
Petroleum jelly	1/2 cup
Water	1/2 cup

☞ Dissolve the boric acid, lanolin, and petroleum jelly over low heat. Add the glycerin and water.

LAVENDER HAND LOTION

Alcohol	1/2 cup
Witch hazel	1/2 cup
Glycerin	2 tablespoons
Camphor	1/2 teaspoon
Oil of lavender	1/4 teaspoon

☞ Dissolve the oil and the camphor in 1/4 cup of the alcohol. Add the rest of the alcohol and the remaining ingredients. Shake well to mix.

LEMON HAND LOTION [1]

Tincture of green soap	1 tablespoon
Glycerin	2 tablespoons
Camphor	1/2 teaspoon
Alcohol	1/4 cup
Water	1 cup
Oil of lemon	1 teaspoon

☞ Dissolve the camphor and oil in the alcohol. Add the remaining ingredients.

LEMON HAND LOTION [2]

Boric acid powder	1/4 teaspoon
Glycerin	1 tablespoon
Alcohol	1/4 cup
Water	1/3 cup
Oil of lemon	1/2 teaspoon

☞ Dissolve the boric acid and the oil in the alcohol, and add the remaining ingredients.

NEROLI HAND LOTION

Soap flakes	3 tablespoons
Lanolin	4 tablespoons
Borax	1/4 teaspoon
Water	1 cup
Oil of neroli	1/4 teaspoon

☞ Dissolve the borax and the soap in 1/2 cup of water. Melt the lanolin in the rest of water over low heat, and add to the first mixture. Stir in the oil of neroli.

PUERTO RICO HAND LOTION

Alcohol	2 tablespoons
Rum	1 tablespoon
Glycerin	3 tablespoons
Tragacanth	1 teaspoon
Water, hot	1 cup
Oil of bay	1/4 teaspoon

☞ Soak the tragacanth in the water to form a mucilage. Add the remaining ingredients.

QUINCE-SEED HAND LOTION

Quince seeds	1 teaspoon
Water, hot	1 cup
Alcohol	1 tablespoon
Glycerin	2 tablespoons

☞ Soak the quince seeds in the water to form a mucilage. Strain, then add the remaining ingredients.

ROSEWATER HAND LOTION

Alcohol	1/4 cup
Tragacanth	2 teaspoons
Tincture of benzoin	1/4 teaspoon
Glycerin	2 tablespoons
Rosewater	1/4 cup
Water	1 1/4 cups

☞ Soak the tragacanth in the water to form a mucilage. Add the other ingredients.

WITCH HAZEL HAND LOTION

Tincture of benzoin	1/2 teaspoon
Camphor	1/4 teaspoon
Alcohol	2 tablespoons
Glycerin	2 tablespoons
Witch hazel	1 cup

☞ Dissolve the camphor in the alcohol.   Add the other ingredients.

LEMON–WITCH HAZEL HAND LOTION

Alcohol	1/2 cup
Camphor	1 teaspoon
Witch hazel	1/4 cup
Oil of lemon	1/2 teaspoon

☞ Dissolve the oil and camphor in the alcohol.   Add the witch hazel.

CHAPPED SKIN LOTION

Glycerin	1/2 cup
Water	1/2 cup
Rosewater	1/2 cup

☞ Combine the ingredients.

DRY SKIN LOTION

Borax	1 teaspoon
Glycerin	3/4 cup
Water	1/2 cup

☞ Dissolve the borax in the water.   Add the glycerin.

OILY SKIN LOTION

Camphor	2 teaspoons
Alcohol	1/3 cup

| Glycerin | 1 tablespoon |
| Water | 1 cup |

☞ Dissolve the camphor in the alcohol. Add the glycerin and the water.

OILY SKIN ROSE LOTION

Boric acid powder	2 teaspoons
Alcohol	1 tablespoon
Rosewater	1/2 cup

☞ Dissolve the boric acid in the alcohol. Add the rosewater.

LEMON FACE LOTION

Boric acid powder	1 tablespoon
Glycerin	2 tablespoons
Menthol	1/2 teaspoon
Oil of lemon	1/2 teaspoon
Alcohol	1 cup
Witch hazel	1/4 cup
Rosewater	1/4 cup

☞ Dissolve the menthol, boric acid, and oil of lemon in the alcohol. Add the remaining ingredients.

ORANGE-FLOWER FACE LOTION

Potassium carbonate	3 tablespoons
Water	1 1/4 cups
Orange-flower water	1/2 cup plus 2 tablespoons
Alcohol	1 tablespoon

☞ Dissolve the potassium carbonate in the water. Add the orange-flower water and the alcohol.

CREAMS

ALMOND HAND CREAM

White beeswax	1/2 cup
Quince seeds	1/2 teaspoon
Water, hot	1/2 cup
Stearic acid	3/4 cup
Borax	1/2 teaspoon
Glycerin	1 tablespoon
Alcohol	1 tablespoon
Oil of sweet almond	1/4 teaspoon

☞ Soak the quince seeds in the water to form a mucilage. Melt the beeswax, stearic acid, and borax together over low heat. Stir the mucilage into the melted wax mixture. Dissolve the oil in the alcohol, and add the glycerin. Combine the two mixtures.

LILY HAND CREAM

Lily of the valley flowers, crushed	1 cup
Rendered fat, any kind	1 cup
Wine, white, any kind	1 cup

☞ Combine the lily of the valley flowers and the wine in a bottle. Cover, and let set for three days. Melt the fat over low heat. Strain the wine, and stir gradually into the fat.

ROSE HAND CREAM

Tincture of benzoin	1 tablespoon
Glycerin	1 tablespoon
Camphor	1 teaspoon
Witch hazel	2 tablespoons
Rosewater	2 tablespoons

☞ Dissolve the camphor in the witch hazel. Add the remaining ingredients.

ELDER-FLOWER FACE CREAM

Rendered fat	1 cup
Mutton suet	2 tablespoons
Elder-flower water	1 cup
Tincture of benzoin	1 tablespoon
Oil of rosemary	1 teaspoon

☞ Melt the fat and suet together over low heat. Add the elder-flower water and simmer on lowest heat for 30 minutes. Take from the heat and let set overnight. In the morning, pour off the water that has floated to the top. Reheat, and add the oil of rosemary. When cool, add the tincture of benzoin.

VENUS FACE CREAM

White wax	1/3 cup
Stearic acid	1 tablespoon
Castor oil	1 cup
Glycerin	1/4 cup
Precipitated sulfur	1 teaspoon
Water	1 tablespoon

☞ Melt the wax and the stearic acid over low heat. Add the sulfur and stir until it dissolves. Stir in the glycerin and the water. Add the castor oil gradually.

ALMOND SKIN CREAM

Almonds, sliced	1/4 cup
Borax	1 teaspoon
Glycerin	1/4 cup
Cologne water	1 teaspoon
Rosewater	1/2 cup

☞ Combine the almonds, borax, and rosewater in a blender. Add the glycerin and cologne water.

GLYCERIN HONEY SKIN CREAM

Liquid soap	1 1/2 teaspoons
Water	2 tablespoons
Glycerin	3/4 cup
Honey	2 tablespoons

☞ Combine the ingredients.

GLYCERIN SKIN CREAM

Liquid soap	1 teaspoon
Water	1/4 cup
Glycerin	1 cup

☞ Combine the ingredients.

LANOLIN SKIN CREAM

Petroleum jelly	3/4 cup
Paraffin	2 tablespoons
Lanolin	2 tablespoons
Water	2 tablespoons

☞ Melt the petroleum jelly, paraffin, and lanolin over low heat. Gradually stir in the water.

LANOLIN AND COCOA BUTTER SKIN CREAM

Lanolin	2 tablespoons
Cocoa butter	1 1/2 tablespoons
Peanut oil	2 tablespoons
Oil of bitter almond	1/2 teaspoon
Water	1/2 cup

☞ Melt the lanolin and cocoa butter together. Stir in the peanut oil and oil of bitter almond. Add the water, in a steady stream, stirring constantly.

LIQUID LANOLIN SKIN CREAM

Liquid soap	1 teaspoon
Water	1/2 cup
Lanolin	3 tablespoons
Glycerin	3 tablespoons

☞ Melt the lanolin over low heat. Stir in the glycerin and the water. Add the soap.

BABY SKIN CREAM

Alcohol	1 tablespoon
Mineral oil	1 tablespoon

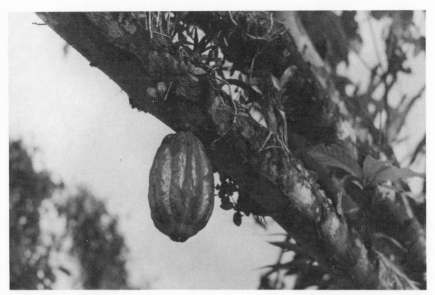

In the cocoa pod are beans from which cocoa butter is expressed for use in creams and lotions. (Theobroma cacao) U.S. Department of Agriculture.

Lanolin	2 teaspoons
Petroleum jelly	1/4 cup
Glycerin	2 teaspoons
Rosewater	1/4 cup

☞ Melt the lanolin and the petroleum jelly together over low heat. Stir in the mineral oil. Add the glycerin and the rosewater. Let cool, and stir in the alcohol.

CONDITIONERS

GLYCERIN-LANOLIN HAND CONDITIONER

Boric acid powder	1 teaspoon
Glycerin	1 1/2 tablespoons
Lanolin	1 1/2 tablespoons
Petroleum jelly	3 tablespoons

☞ Dissolve the boric acid, lanolin, and petroleum jelly over low heat. Stir in the glycerin.

GLYCERIN VIOLET HAND CONDITIONER

Liquid soap	1/4 cup
Orrisroot powder	3 tablespoons
Cornstarch	3 tablespoons
Glycerin	1/3 cup
Oil of neroli	1/4 teaspoon
Oil of lemon	1/2 teaspoon

☛ Combine the orrisroot, cornstarch, and glycerin. Stir in the soap and oils.

HONEY-ALMOND HAND CONDITIONER

Honey	1 tablespoon
Liquid soap	2 teaspoons
Almond oil	1/4 cup
Oil of orange	1/2 teaspoon
Boric acid powder	1/2 teaspoon

☛ Combine the boric acid with the honey, and stir in the oils. When they are well mixed, add the soap.

WHEAT-ALMOND HAND CONDITIONER

Wheat flour	1/2 cup
Almond meal	2 tablespoons
Orrisroot powder	1 tablespoon
Extract of orange	2 tablespoons
Glycerin	1 tablespoon

☛ Mix the first three ingredients together. Add the extract and the glycerin, and mix to a smooth paste.

WHEAT-ALMOND SKIN CONDITIONER

Wheat flour	1 cup
Almonds, ground to a powder	1/4 cup
Orrisroot powder	2 tablespoons
Glycerin	1 tablespoon
Alcohol	2 tablespoons
Oil of rose	5 drops

☛ Mix the ingredients to a smooth paste. To use, mix two tablespoons of the mixture with one tablespoon of water.

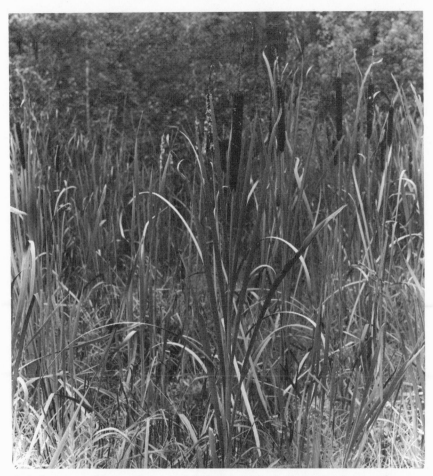

Cattails are emollient and are used in facial masks, bath preparations, and creams. They grow in damp, low areas. (Typha latifolia) Arnold Krochmal.

HONEY GLYCERIN SKIN CONDITIONER

Gelatin	1 tablespoon
Water	1/4 cup
Honey	1/2 cup
Glycerin	1 cup
Boric acid powder	1 teaspoon

Soak the gelatin in the water for five minutes to soften, and then dissolve it over low heat. Add the boric acid, and continue heating until the boric acid is dissolved. Combine the honey and glycerin, and add to the gelatin mixture.

SOME EMOLLIENT PLANTS

Name	Part Used	Botanical Name
Cattail	Root	*Typha*
Fig	Fruit	*Ficus*
Groundsel	Leaves	*Senecio*
Jimson weed	Seeds	*Datura*
Locust	Flowers	*Robinia*
Lotus	Root, leaves, seeds	*Nelumbo*
Mallow	Foliage	*Malva*
Ragweed	Foliage	*Ambrosia*
Rose mallow	Seeds (also astringent)	*Hibiscus*
Water shield	Root	*Brasenia*

Massage Creams

The Egyptians, Romans, and Greeks used massage creams and oils in the spa-like baths, exercise rooms, and massage parlors they frequented. The Greeks considered massage creams essential during vigorous training for the Olympic games, which of course they originated. The medicated ingredients used, including menthol, camphor, and eucalyptus, were then, as now, quite soothing to the muscles; they relieved soreness, aches, and pains as well as stimulating muscle tone.

The Greeks used massage before going into battle to prepare the body for the physical strain of warfare. Today athletes, home gardeners, housewives, and many other people use it to relieve physical strain and stress.

CAMPHOR MASSAGE CREAM

Camphor	1/2 teaspoon
Mineral oil	1/4 cup
Alcohol	2 tablespoons plus 1 teaspoon
Water, warm	2 tablespoons

☛ Dissolve the camphor in the alcohol. Stir in the water. Add the mineral oil.

GLYCERIN MASSAGE CREAM

Irish moss	1 tablespoon
Water	1 1/4 cups
Glycerin	1/4 cup
Boric acid powder	1/2 teaspoon
Cologne	2 tablespoons

☛ Dissolve the glycerin and boric acid in two tablespoons of water. Boil the Irish moss gently in the remaining water for 10 minutes to form a mucilage. Combine the two mixtures. Cool and add the cologne.

MEDICATED MASSAGE CREAM

Menthol	1/4 teaspoon
Camphor	1 teaspoon
Oil of eucalyptus	1/2 teaspoon
Petroleum jelly	1 cup

☛ Melt the petroleum jelly over low heat. Add the remaining ingredients, and stir until the menthol and camphor dissolve.

MENTHOL MASSAGE CREAM

Menthol	1/4 teaspoon
Tragacanth	1 tablespoon
Glycerin	2 teaspoons
Alcohol	1 tablespoon
Water, hot	2 1/2 cups

☛ Soak the tragacanth in one cup of the water to form a mucilage. Dissolve the menthol in the alcohol, and add the glycerin. Combine the mixtures and stir in the remaining water.

WITCH HAZEL MASSAGE CREAM

Lanolin	1/4 cup
Petroleum jelly	2 tablespoons
Witch hazel	2 teaspoons

☛ Warm the witch hazel over a water bath. Add the lanolin and the petroleum jelly, and heat gently until melted.

MASSAGE OIL

Lanolin	1 1/2 tablespoons
Olive oil	1 cup

☛ Melt the lanolin. Add to the warmed olive oil.

Nail Preparations

Proper nail care requires the use of enamels, polishes, polish removers, and cuticle softeners and removers. Since nail polishes and polish removers require sophisticated chemical formulas, they are not included here.

Cuticle softeners and creams aid in keeping the cuticles soft and supple, and add to the general appearance of the nails by helping keep the cuticles neat.

CUTICLE CREAM

Beeswax	1 teaspoon
Liquid soap	1 tablespoon
Paraffin	1/2 cup

☛ Melt the beeswax and paraffin over low heat. Stir in the soap.

CUTICLE ICE

Menthol	1/4 teaspoon
Paraffin	1/4 cup
Petroleum jelly	1/4 cup

☛ Melt the paraffin with the petroleum jelly over low heat. Add the menthol and stir until dissolved.

NAIL OINTMENT

Petroleum jelly	1/4 cup
Soap flakes	1 teaspoon
Oil of bergamot	5 drops

☛ Melt the jelly over low heat. Add the soap and the oil.

ALMOND CUTICLE SOFTENER

Olive oil	1 cup
Petroleum jelly	3 tablespoons
Oil of sweet almond	1/8 teaspoon

☞ Melt the petroleum jelly over low heat and add the olive oil. Stir in the oil.

MENTHOL CUTICLE SOFTENER

Petroleum jelly	1/2 cup
Paraffin	2 teaspoons
Menthol	1/2 teaspoon
Thymol	1/8 teaspoon

☞ Melt the paraffin and the petroleum jelly together over low heat. Add the menthol and thymol.

LANOLIN CUTICLE CREAM

Lanolin	1 tablespoon
Paraffin	1/2 cup

☞ Melt over low heat.

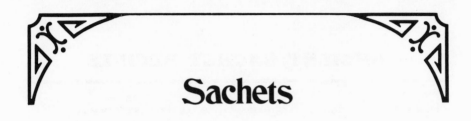

Sachets

The Egyptians washed their walls with rosewater; the Romans scattered rose petals on the floor, and had fountains of rosewater. These ways of scenting the air were the beginnings of sachets, whose purpose is to pleasantly perfume a person's clothing and surroundings.

In the past the choice of a particular sachet scent has been a fad or a fashion of the time. In England, lavender sachets were used in bedding as well as other linen and clothes. The most popular scent has been potpourri, a grand mixture of several aromatic plants. But there are enough varieties to suit everyone's taste.

Table salt or sand is often added to a sachet to provide bulk, but is not necessary. Orrisroot, also used, is a fixative. It is necessary to let any sachet set for about two weeks so that the scents may mingle and stabilize before packaging.

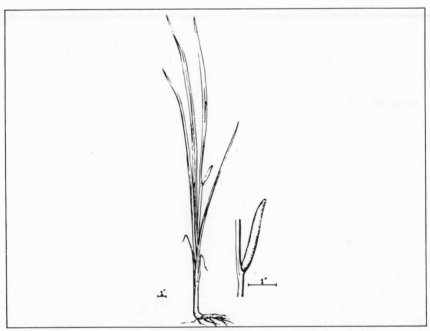

Sweet flag is a moisture- and water-loving plant whose highly aromatic roots are used in sachets. (Acorus calamus) U.S. Forest Service.

ANCIENT SACHET RECIPES

"Powders of Callamus, orris, roses, white sanders (sandalwood), Beni-mym (benzoin), Cypres, Violette, and Spyke. Mingle together."

"A violette Powder for the perfuming of linen used by the King Henry of France" consisted of "orris root, rose leaves, sandalwood, cypres, bengamen, marjoleine, storax, calamus, giroffle, ambergris, coriander, and lavender."

A sachet powder of Queen Isabella of Spain recorded in a French manuscript of 1631: "rose leaves, orris root, calamus, storax, benzoin, girofle flowers, and coriander."

Taken from a manuscript of the 16th century: "To make a sweet powder for Bagges. Take Damask rose leaves, orris root, calamith, benzoin gum, and make into a powder and fill ye bags."

ACACIA SHOWER-OF-GOLD SACHET

Cassie flowers	6 cups
Orrisroot powder	6 tablespoons
Salt	1 cup

☞ Combine the ingredients.

ACACIA SACHET

Cassie flowers	4 cups
Orrisroot powder	1/4 cup
Starch	1/2 cup

☞ Combine the ingredients.

CEYLON SACHET

Rose leaves	2 cups
Vetiver root	1 3/4 cups
Patchouly herb	1 1/2 cups
Mace	3/4 cup

☞ Combine the ingredients.

CEYLON SACHET POWDER

Mace	1 tablespoon
Patchouly herb	2 tablespoons
Vetiver root	1/4 cup
Rose leaves	1 1/2 cups

☞ Mix the ingredients and grind to a powder.

CLOVE-TRILISA SACHET POWDER

Orrisroot	1/4 cup
Lavender flowers	4 cups
Patchouly herb	2 cups
Ground cloves	1/4 cup
Deerstongue leaves	1 cup
Ground allspice	1/2 cup
Oil of rose	10 drops
Oil of lavender	10 drops
Oil of neroli	12 drops
Oil of sandalwood	1/4 teaspoon

☞ Mix the dry ingredients together and add the oils.

CYPRIAN SACHET POWDER

Cedarwood chips	1/2 cup
Rhodium chips	1/2 cup
Sandalwood chips	1/2 cup
Oil of rhodium	7 drops

☞ Grind the woods to a powder. Add the oils.

FLOWERS SACHET

Calamus root	3/4 cup
Caraway seed	1/2 cup
Ground cloves	1/4 cup
Lavender flowers	2 cups
Marjoram	1 cup
Mint	1 cup
Rose leaves	2 cups
Rosemary	1/2 cup
Thyme	1/4 cup

☞ Combine the ingredients.

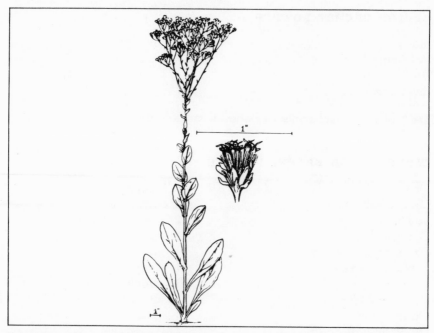

Deerstongue is a wild perennial whose vanilla-smelling foliage is harvested in Florida and Georgia and used in sachets and facial preparations. It is also a flavoring for cigars and pipe tobacco. (Trilisa odoratissima) U.S. Forest Service.

FLOWERS-OF-THE-FIELD SACHET POWDER

Calamus root	1 cup
Lavender flowers	2 cups
Rose petals	2 cups
Caraway seed	1/4 cup
Marjoram	1/4 cup
Mint	1/2 cup
Thyme	1/4 cup
Rosemary	1/4 cup
Ground cloves	1 tablespoon

☞ Grind all ingredients to a fine powder.

FRANGIPANI SACHET

Orrisroot powder	1/2 cup
Rose petals	5 cups
Vanilla bean	1

Benzoin	2 tablespoons
Oil of sandalwood	10 drops
Oil of neroli	9 drops
Oil of lavender	5 drops
Oil of bergamot	7 drops
Oil of cassie	1/8 teaspoon
Oil of pimento	4 drops
Oil of rose	1/8 teaspoon

☞ Mix the dry ingredients together before adding the oils.

INDIAN SACHET POWDER

Sandalwood	1/4 cup
Orrisroot powder	3/4 cup
Ground cinnamon	1 cup
Ground cloves	2 tablespoons
Oil of rose	10 drops
Oil of lavender	10 drops

☞ Mix the dry ingredients and grind to a powder. Add the oils.

INDIAN SACHET

Orrisroot powder	1 cup
Ground cinnamon	1/2 cup
Sandalwood	2 cups
Oil of clove	1/8 teaspoon
Oil of rose	1/8 teaspoon
Oil of lavender	10 drops

☞ Combine the ingredients.

LAVENDER SACHET

Lavender flowers	4 cups
Benzoin	2 tablespoons
Oil of lavender	1 teaspoon

☞ Grind the benzoin to a powder. Put in a mixing bowl and combine with the oil. Add the lavender flowers.

LAVENDER-BERGAMOT SACHET

Lavender flowers	4 cups
Benzoin	1 1/2 tablespoons
Oil of bergamot	1/4 teaspoon
Oil of lavender	1 teaspoon

☞ Grind the benzoin to a powder, and add the oils. Mix with the flowers.

LAVENDER SACHET POWDER

Lavender flowers	5 cups
Benzoin	1/4 cup
Oil of lavender	1 teaspoon
Oil of rose	1/8 teaspoon

☞ Grind the lavender flowers and benzoin together. Add the oils.

LEMON SACHET

Lemon peel, cubed and dried	1/2 cup
Lavender flowers	3 cups
Orrisroot powder	1/4 cup
Rosemary	1 cup
Oil of lemon	1/2 teaspoon

☞ Combine the ingredients.

MEDITERRANEAN SACHET POWDER

Benzoin	1/2 cup
Sandalwood	3/4 cup
Thyme	1 cup
Orrisroot powder	3/4 cup
Vetiver root	1 1/2 cups
Oil of rose geranium	1/8 teaspoon

☞ Grind the dry ingredients to a powder. Add the oil.

ORANGE SACHET

Orange peels, cubed and dried	2 cups
Lemon peels, cubed and dried	1 cup
Orrisroot	1/2 cup
Ground cinnamon	1/4 cup
Oil of lemon grass	1/8 teaspoon
Oil of orange	1/2 teaspoon
Oil of neroli	1/8 teaspoon

☞ Combine the orange and lemon peels, orrisroot, and cinnamon. Add the oils.

PATCHOULY-ROSEWOOD SACHET

Patchouly herb	4 cups
Orrisroot powder	1/2 cup
Rosewood	1/4 cup
Benzoin	2 tablespoons
Oil of patchouly	1 teaspoon
Oil of rose	5 drops

☞ Combine the patchouly herb, orrisroot, and rosewood. Add the benzoin and the oils.

PATCHOULY SACHET

Patchouly herb	2 cups
Orrisroot powder	1/4 cup
Oil of patchouly	12 drops
Oil of rose geranium	12 drops

☞ Combine the orrisroot and patchouly herb. Add the oils and mix well.

PERSIAN SACHET

Orrisroot powder	1/2 cup
Rose leaves	3 cups
Tonka bean	1 teaspoon
Oil of cinnamon	10 drops
Oil of nutmeg	1/8 teaspoon
Oil of rose	1/8 teaspoon
Oil of cloves	1/8 teaspoon

☞ Combine the ingredients.

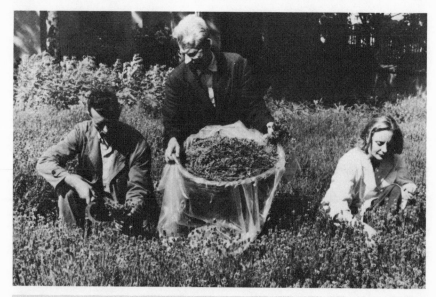

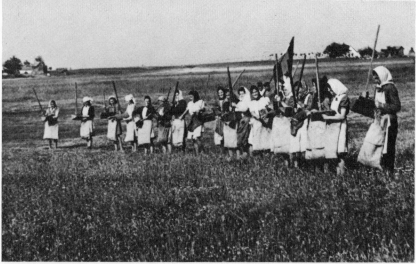

Wild plants are important to the agriculture of Yugoslavia because of their use in the cosmetic industry. In the upper photo, wild lavender is being harvested. In the bottom photo, peasant women are harvesting chamomile. Dr. Jovan Tucakov, Director, Institute of Pharmacognosy, Belgrade, Yugoslavia.

PORTUGAL POWDER

Lemon peels, dried and ground	3/4 cup
Orange peels, dried and ground	1 1/2 cups
Orrisroot powder	3/4 cup
Ground cinnamon	1/4 cup
Oil of lemon grass	10 drops
Oil of neroli	10 drops
Oil of orange	1 teaspoon

☛ Grind the peels to a powder, and combine with the orrisroot and cinnamon. Add the oils.

POTPOURRI SACHET POWDER [1]

Rose leaves	3 cups
Lavender flowers	3 cups
Orrisroot, ground to a coarse powder	1/4 cup
Whole cloves	2 tablespoons
Ground cinnamon	2 tablespoons
Ground allspice	2 tablespoons
Salt	1/2 cup

☛ Combine the ingredients.

POTPOURRI SACHET POWDER [2]

Lavender flowers	3 cups
Whole cloves	1/4 cup
Ground allspice	1/4 cup
Rose leaves	2 cups
Reseda	1/4 cup
Orrisroot powder	1/2 cup
Vanilla	1 bean
Ground cinnamon	1/2 cup
Table salt	1/2 cup

☛ Combine the ingredients.

POTPOURRI SACHET POWDER [3]

Rose leaves	3 cups
Lavender flowers	3 cups
Reseda	1/2 cup
Vanilla bean, ground	1 teaspoon
Salt	1 cup
Orrisroot powder	1/2 cup
Ground cloves	1/4 cup
Ground cinnamon	1/4 cup
Ground allspice	1/4 cup

☞ Grind the rose leaves, lavender flowers, and the reseda to a powder. Combine with the other ingredients.

ROSE-SANDALWOOD SACHET POWDER

Rose leaves	4 cups
Sandalwood	1/2 cup
Oil of rose	1 teaspoon

☞ Grind the rose leaves and the sandalwood to a powder. Add the oil of rose.

ROSE SACHET POWDER

Rose geranium herb	1/4 cup
Rose leaves	4 cups
Sandalwood	1/2 cup
Oil of rose	1 teaspoon

☞ Grind the dry ingredients to a powder. Add the oil.

ROSE SACHET

Rose petals	4 cups
Rose leaves	1 cup
Sandalwood, crushed	1 cup
Salt	1/2 cup
Oil of rose	1 tablespoon

☞ Combine the ingredients.

SPICED SACHET POWDER

Orrisroot powder	1/2 cup
Starch	2 cups
Oil of sandalwood	1/2 teaspoon
Oil of bergamot	1/4 teaspoon
Oil of neroli	1/8 teaspoon

☞ Combine the orrisroot and starch. Add the oils.

VERBENA SACHET POWDER

Lemon peels, sliced and dried	1 cup
Orange peels, sliced and dried	1 cup
Caraway seed	1/4 cup
Oil of verbena	10 drops
Oil of lemon	10 drops
Oil of bergamot	1/8 teaspoon

☞ Blend the peels and caraway seed to a fine powder. Add the oils.

PERFUMED SACHET TABLET

Paraffin	1 cup
Oil of bergamot	1 teaspoon
Oil of lavender	1 teaspoon
Oil of cloves	1/2 teaspoon
Oil of rose geranium	10 drops
Vanilla extract	1 teaspoon

☞ Melt the paraffin over water. Let it cool a little, then stir in the oils and the extract. Pour into small molds.

Shaving Preparations

Shaving creams, soaps, and shaving milks all serve to make the chore of shaving less damaging to men's faces and dispositions by softening the beard and helping the razor slide over the face.

Some of the liquid formulas I have listed require shaking before use. I have found that those which tend to separate can be combined in a blender. Liquids and semi-liquids should be stored in wide-mouthed containers, which will accommodate a shaving brush more easily; these can also be rubbed on.

Shaving powders should be mixed with one tablespoonful of warm water and applied with a brush.

After-shave lotions have two purposes. One is to help heal cuts, abrasions, and nicked areas. The other is to refresh the shaver's skin and leave it sweet smelling. All are mildly astringent, containing 40–60 percent alcohol. However, I have included formulas for non-alcoholic after-shave creams and lotions.

Talc helps to repair and cover scrapes, nicks, and scratches, covers shiny skin surfaces of those who shave very closely, and leaves a pleasant smell.

SHAVING PREPARATIONS

ALMOND SHAVING MILK

Almond oil	1 1/2 tablespoons
Glycerin	1/4 cup
Gum arabic	1 tablespoon
Rosewater	1 cup
Tincture of benzoin	1/3 cup

☛ Combine the almond oil, glycerin, gum arabic, and rosewater in a blender to form an emulsion; then add the tincture of benzoin.

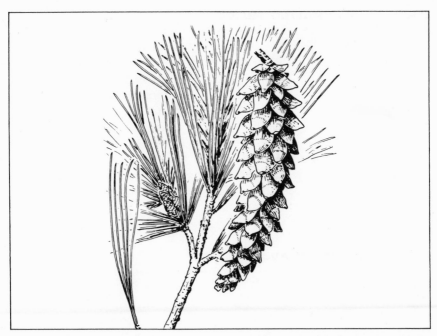

The white pine is one of the sources of pine-needle oil used in bath preparations, shaving lotions, and soaps. (Pinus strobus) University of West Virginia.

CAMPHOR SHAVING MILK

Camphor	1/4 teaspoon
Glycerin	1 tablespoon
Oil of lavender	1/2 teaspoon
Alcohol	1/4 cup plus 2 tablespoons
Borax	1 tablespoon
Water	1 1/4 cups
Lemon juice	3 tablespoons

☞ Dissolve the camphor and the oil in the alcohol. Add the other ingredients, and shake well to mix.

CITRUS SHAVING MILK

Lanolin	1 teaspoon
Borax	1/4 teaspoon
Glycerin	1 tablespoon
Orange-flower water	2 1/2 tablespoons
Rosewater	2 1/2 tablespoons
Tincture of benzoin	2 teaspoons

☞ Melt the lanolin and the borax over low heat. Stir in the other ingredients.

COCONUT OIL SHAVING MILK

Lanolin	3 tablespoons
Coconut oil	2 tablespoons
Borax	1 tablespoon
Soap flakes	3 tablespoons
Water	2 cups
Rosewater	1 cup

☞ Melt the coconut oil and lanolin together over low heat. Set aside. Heat the water, and add the borax and soap. Stir until dissolved. Add to the coconut oil and lanolin. Stir in the rosewater.

LEMON SHAVING POWDER

Soap flakes	3 cups
Cornstarch	1/4 cup
Sodium carbonate	3 tablespoons
Oil of lemon	1 teaspoon

☞ Combine the dry ingredients and then add the oil.

LIME SHAVING POWDER

Soap flakes	1 cup
Rice flour	2 tablespoons
Mineral oil	1 tablespoon
Boric acid powder	2 teaspoons
Oil of lime	1/2 teaspoon

☞ Combine the dry ingredients and then stir in the oils.

COCOA BUTTER SHAVING CREAM

Stearic acid	1/4 cup
Cocoa butter	1 tablespoon
Sodium carbonate	1 tablespoon
Borax	2 tablespoons
Glycerin	1/4 cup

| Alcohol | 2 tablespoons |
| Water, hot | 1 3/4 cups |

☞ Dissolve the sodium carbonate, borax, and glycerin in the hot water. Melt the stearic acid and cocoa butter over low heat, and add the water solution. Stir briskly until a smooth white soapy mixture is formed. Continue stirring until cool, and then add the alcohol.

UNSCENTED SHAVING CREAM [1]

Stearic acid	1/4 cup
Ammonia	2 teaspoons
Borax	1 teaspoon
Water, hot	1 cup
Soap flakes	2 tablespoons

☞ Dissolve the borax and soap in the water. Melt the stearic acid over low heat, and pour into the water mixture in a steady stream. When the mixture cools, stir in the ammonia.

UNSCENTED SHAVING CREAM [2]

Stearic acid	1/4 cup
Mineral oil	1/4 cup
Paraffin	1/4 cup plus 2 tablespoons
Soap flakes	1/4 cup
Water, hot	1 cup

☞ Dissolve the soap in the water. Melt the stearic acid and the paraffin together over low heat, and stir into the water mixture. When well mixed, stir in the mineral oil.

COCOA BUTTER SHAVING SOAP

Soap flakes	3 tablespoons
Water	1/2 cup
Cocoa butter	1 tablespoon
Tincture of benzoin	1 teaspoon
Oil of bitter almond	5 drops
Glycerin	2 tablespoons

☞ Dissolve the soap in the water. Melt the cocoa butter, and add the water mixture. Add the remaining ingredients. Blend in a blender until the mixture emulsifies.

AFTER SHAVE

ALMOND CREAM AFTER-SHAVE

Tragacanth	1 teaspoon
Glycerin	1/4 cup
Borax	1/4 cup
Water, hot	1 1/2 cups
Oil of bitter almond	1 teaspoon

☞ Soak the tragacanth in the water to form a mucilage. Add the glycerin and borax. Stir in the oil.

ASTRINGENT AFTER-SHAVE

Alum	1 teaspoon
Menthol	1/4 teaspoon
Camphor	1/4 teaspoon
Boric acid powder	1/2 teaspoon
Glycerin	1 tablespoon
Alcohol	1/3 cup
Water	1 1/2 cups

☞ Dissolve the first four ingredients in the alcohol. Add the glycerin and the water. Let set several days until it clears.

CAMDEN AFTER-SHAVE

Menthol	1/4 teaspoon
Boric acid powder	1 teaspoon
Glycerin	1 teaspoon
Alcohol	1/2 cup
Water	1 cup

☞ Dissolve the menthol and boric acid in the alcohol. Add the glycerin and water. Shake well. Let set for several days until it clears.

HUNTSMAN AFTER-SHAVE

Boric acid powder	1 1/2 teaspoons
Alcohol	1 tablespoon
Tincture of benzoin	2 teaspoons
Glycerin	1 tablespoon
Witch hazel	1/2 cup
Water	3/4 cup

☞ Dissolve the boric acid in the alcohol. Add the remaining ingredients and shake well. Let set for several days until it clears.

MENTHOL AFTER-SHAVE

Tragacanth	1 teaspoon
Glycerin	1/4 cup
Alcohol	3/4 cup
Menthol	1/4 teaspoon
Water, hot	3/4 cup

☞ Combine the tragacanth and water, and let set to form a mucilage. Dissolve the menthol in the alcohol, and add the mucilage. Shake well, then add the glycerin. Let set several days until it clears.

PAMLICO AFTER-SHAVE

Alcohol	1/3 cup
Glycerin	2 teaspoons
Menthol	1/2 teaspoon
Boric acid powder	1 teaspoon
Water	1 cup
Oil of sandalwood	5 drops
Oil of lemon	1/4 teaspoon

☞ Dissolve the menthol, boric acid, and oils in the alcohol. Add the glycerin and water, and shake well. Let set for several days until it clears.

ST. CROIX AFTER-SHAVE

Rum	2 tablespoons
Alcohol	1/2 cup
Glycerin	1 tablespoon
Oil of bay	1 teaspoon
Water	1/3 cup

☞ Dissolve the oil in the alcohol. Add the other ingredients and shake well. Let set several days until it clears.

WEST INDIES AFTER-SHAVE

Alcohol	1/3 cup
Water	1/3 cup
Glycerin	1 tablespoon
Menthol	1/8 teaspoon
Oil of bay	5 drops

☞ Dissolve the oil and menthol in the alcohol. Add the remaining ingredients, and shake well. Let set for several days until it clears.

WITCH HAZEL AFTER-SHAVE

Alum	2 teaspoons
Glycerin	2 tablespoons
Alcohol	1/4 cup
Witch hazel	1 cup
Water	1 cup

☞ Put all the ingredients in a jar. Cover, and shake well to mix. Let set for several days until it clears.

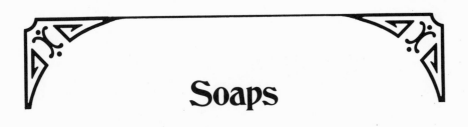

Soaps

Our pioneer ancestors learned to know which native plants would serve as soaps and detergents for their laundry needs. Some of this knowledge came from their own observation and experience, some from watching the Indians.

There are many wild plants growing in all parts of the United States which can be used to produce the suds to clean pots and pans on camping trips, as well as to launder clothes, and are considered particularly useful for shampoos. (See the list on page 180.) I hope the reader will be cautious in trying out these plants as soap substitutes.

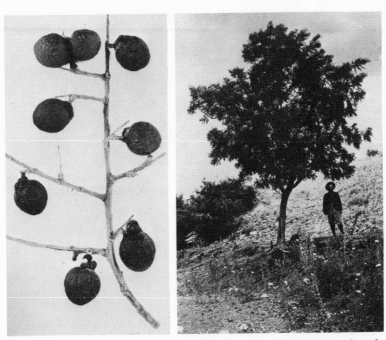

Soapberry species were used as a source of detergents by Indians and early settlers. (left, Sapindus marginates, Florida soapberry; right, S. drummondi, western soapberry) U.S. Forest Service.

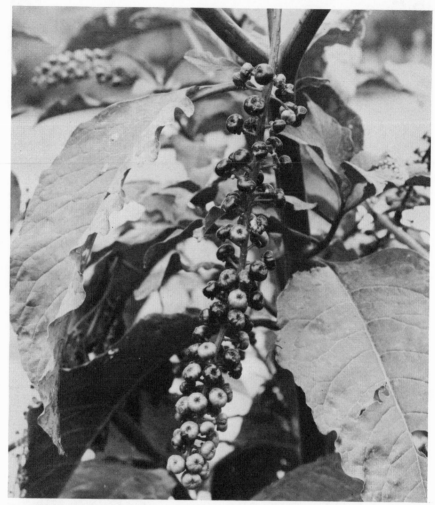

A rapid-growing shrub, the pokeberry is rich in saponins (soaplike substances). The fruits are often used in Appalachia and in Africa to create suds for laundering. (Phytolacca americana) Arnold Krochmal.

So many of our wild plants have been overused in past decades that large numbers of species are threatened with extinction—a sad thought indeed!

Making soap from scratch is a job to do outdoors, requiring materials hard to find in urban areas and necessitating large kettles. I have not given any formulas for soap-making because of these and other difficulties involved.

LIQUID SOAP

Soap flakes	3 tablespoons
Alcohol	1 teaspoon
Water, hot	1 cup
Oil of strawberry	1/8 teaspoon

☞ Dissolve the soap in the water, and dissolve the oil in the alcohol. Combine the two mixtures.

LIQUID GLYCERIN SOAP

Soap flakes	2 tablespoons
Glycerin	1/4 cup
Water, hot	1/2 cup
Alcohol	2 tablespoons
Talc	1 tablespoon

☞ Combine the soap and water. Combine the talc and the alcohol, and stir to a smooth paste. Add the glycerin, and combine with the water mixture.

MEDICATED SOAP

Soap flakes	1/2 cup
Water, hot	1/3 cup
Alcohol	1/2 cup
Potassium carbonate	1/2 cup

☞ Dissolve the potassium carbonate and soap in the water. Add the alcohol.

SOAP SUBSTITUTE

Almond meal	2 tablespoons
Kaolin	2 tablespoons
Borax	1/2 teaspoon
Oil of sweet almond	1/8 teaspoon

☞ Combine the kaolin and borax. Stir in the almond meal and the oil.

SOME PLANTS USED AS SOAP

NAME	PART USED	BOTANICAL NAME
Agave	Root, leaves, stems	*Agave*
Jujube	Fruit	*Zizyphus*
Morning glory	Plant ashes	*Ipomoea*
Ocotillo	Bark, root	*Fouquieria*
Pigweed	Root	*Chenopodium*
Poke	Fruit	*Phytolacca*
Soapberry	Fruit	*Sapindus*
Soap root	Bulb	*Camassia*
Soapwort	Root	*Saponaria*
Spanish bayonet	Root	*Yucca*
Wild gourd	Fruit	*Cucurbita*

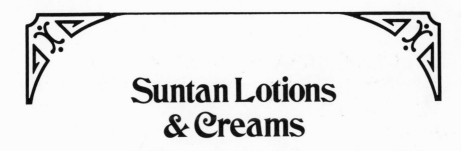

Suntan Lotions & Creams

The first suntan oil was made from the castor oil plant. The Sumerians, and later the Egyptians, rubbed it on the body as a protection against the burning desert sun. Certain tribes in Africa still use palm oil and coconut oil for the same purpose.

The purpose of suntan creams is to promote tanning as well as to prevent burning. There is no mystery or magic to these creams. They are quite simple in composition, and most of those included in this chapter are similar to popular commercial products. Their ingredients are usually cocoa butter, coconut oil, lanolin, sometimes coloring, and scent.

No cream is capable of totally screening the sun's rays. So it is best to use a certain amount of caution and common sense when exposed to the sun, even if you are using a suntan lotion.

ALMOND SUNTAN LOTION

Almonds, sliced	1 tablespoon
Rosewater	1/2 cup
Glycerin	1 tablespoon
Oil of sweet almond	5 drops

☞ Grind the almonds to a smooth paste. Add the glycerin and the oil. Stir until smooth, and gradually add the rosewater, stirring well after each addition.

PALM SUNTAN LOTION

Palm oil	1/4 cup
Coconut oil	1/4 cup
Lanolin	2 tablespoons

☞ Melt the lanolin over a low heat. Stir in the palm and coconut oils.

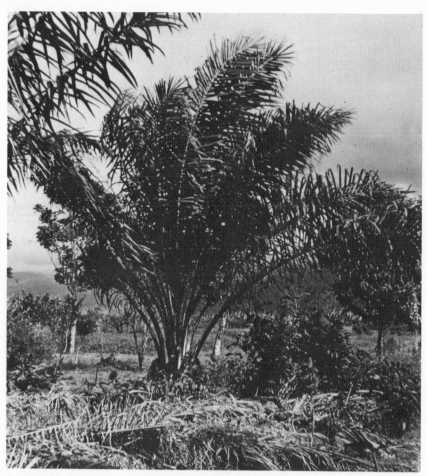

Among the important sources of plant oils, the African oil palm rates high. A tropical tree, it bears a large nutlike fruit on the trunk. This oil palm plantation was photographed on the Pacific coast of Costa Rica. The oil is used in soap manufacture. (Elaeis guineesis) Arnold Krochmal.

TAHITIAN SUNTAN LOTION

Petroleum jelly	1/2 cup
Lanolin	1 tablespoon
Oil of rose	3 drops

☞ Melt the lanolin and petroleum jelly together over low heat. Stir in the oil of rose.

BERGAMOT SUNTAN OIL

Peanut oil	1/4 cup
Olive oil	2 tablespoons
Oil of bergamot	1/4 teaspoon

☞ Combine the ingredients.

JASMINE SUNTAN OIL

Olive oil	1/3 cup
Peanut oil	1/3 cup
Oil of jasmine	1/4 teaspoon

☞ Combine the ingredients.

NEAPOLITAN SUNTAN OIL

Olive oil	1/2 cup
Sesame oil	1 tablespoon
Peanut oil	1/4 cup

☞ Combine the ingredients.

SESAME SUNTAN OIL

Sesame oil	1/2 cup
Olive oil	1/2 cup
Oil of sweet almond	1/4 teaspoon

☞ Combine the ingredients.

SUNFLOWER SUNTAN OIL

Sunflower oil	1/4 cup
Sesame oil	1 teaspoon

☞ Combine the ingredients.

THUJA SUNTAN OIL

Olive oil	1/4 cup
Peanut oil	1/4 cup
Sesame oil	1 teaspoon
Thuja oil	1 1/2 teaspoons
Oil of bergamot	1/4 teaspoon

☞ Combine the ingredients.

Toothpastes, Tooth Powders, Mouth Washes

The original purpose of toothpaste was to keep the teeth clean and the breath inoffensive. Now toothpastes serve these purposes and are also used to protect teeth from decay. The introduction of fluoride into toothpaste is an example of this broadened scope.

Tooth powders and mouth washes have cosmetic, as well as personal health, purposes; they make the breath wholesome and sweet smelling.

TOOTH POWDERS

CARDAMON TOOTH POWDER

Precipitated chalk	1 cup
Soap flakes	1 1/2 tablespoons
Camphor	1/2 teaspoon
Oil of cardamon	1/4 teaspoon

☞ Grind the camphor together with the soap. Add the chalk, and stir in the oil.

CEDARN TOOTH POWDER

Precipitated chalk	2/3 cup
Orrisroot powder	2 tablespoons
Oil of cedarwood	1/2 teaspoon
Oil of peppermint	5 drops

☞ Combine the dry ingredients and then add the oils.

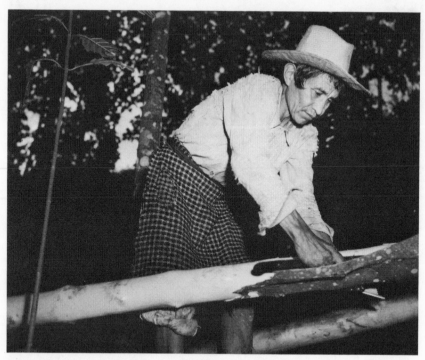

South America is the source of cinchona bark, once the sovereign treatment for malaria. Quinine taken from the bark is used as a preservative in cosmetics. U.S. Department of Agriculture.

CHARCOAL TOOTH POWDER [1]

Powdered charcoal	1/4 cup
Powdered cinchona bark	1 tablespoon
Oil of cloves	1/8 teaspoon
Oil of orange	8 drops

☞ Mix the ingredients.

CHARCOAL TOOTH POWDER [2]

Burnt toast, ground	1/2 cup
Precipitated chalk	1/4 cup

☞ Mix the ingredients.

CLOVE-MINT TOOTH POWDER

Calcium carbonate	3/4 cup
Magnesium carbonate	1 tablespoon
Precipitated chalk	1/4 cup
Borax	2 tablespoons
Oil of cloves	1/8 teaspoon
Oil of peppermint	1/4 teaspoon

☞ Combine the calcium carbonate, magnesium carbonate, chalk, and borax. Add the oils, and mix well.

KITCHEN TOOTH POWDER

Cream of tartar	1/2 cup
Powdered charcoal	1/4 cup
Alum	2 tablespoons
Powdered sugar	1 tablespoon
Oil of cinnamon	1/2 teaspoon

☞ Combine the cream of tartar, charcoal, alum, and sugar. Add the oil.

LEMON TOOTH POWDER

Calcium carbonate	1/4 cup
Magnesium carbonate	2 tablespoons
Orrisroot powder	1 tablespoon
Soap flakes	2 tablespoons
Powdered sugar	1 tablespoon
Oil of lemon	1/4 teaspoon
Thymol	1/8 teaspoon

☞ Combine the dry ingredients, and stir in the oil and the thymol.

LICORICE TOOTH POWDER

Precipitated chalk	1 cup
Soap flakes	1 tablespoon
Licorice-root powder	1 tablespoon

☞ Mix all the ingredients.

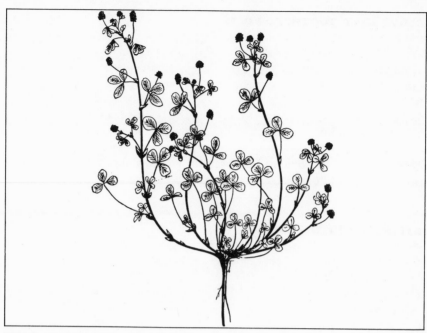

Wild licorice occurs in several species. Licorice is used as a flavoring in tooth-pastes, tooth powders, and mouth washes. This perennial shrublike plant is found in the western and central United States. (Glycyrrhiza spp.) University of Arizona.

LIME TOOTH POWDER

Precipitated chalk	1 cup
Oil of peppermint	2 teaspoons
Oil of lime	1/4 teaspoon

☞ Mix all the ingredients.

MINT TOOTH POWDER

Lactose	1/2 cup
Precipitated chalk	1/2 cup
Oil of peppermint	1/4 teaspoon

☞ Mix the dry ingredients and then add the oil.

ORANGE TOOTH POWDER

Precipitated chalk	1 cup
Orrisroot powder	1/4 cup

| Oil of orange | 1/2 teaspoon |
| Oil of cinnamon | 1/4 teaspoon |

☞ Combine the chalk and the orrisroot, then add the oils.

PEPPERMINT TOOTH POWDER

Precipitated chalk	2/3 cup
Magnesium carbonate	1/4 cup
Soap flakes	1/4 cup
Powdered sugar	2 tablespoons
Oil of peppermint	1/4 teaspoon

☞ Combine the dry ingredients, then add the oil.

SPEARMINT TOOTH POWDER

Precipitated chalk	1 cup
Orrisroot powder	1/4 cup
Powdered sugar	2 teaspoons
Soap flakes	1 teaspoon
Oil of spearmint	1/4 teaspoon

☞ Combine the dry ingredients, then add the oil.

SPICED TOOTH POWDER [1]

Precipitated chalk	1 cup
Orrisroot powder	1/4 cup
Oil of sandalwood	1/4 teaspoon
Oil of cinnamon	1/8 teaspoon

☞ Combine the dry ingredients, then add the oil.

SPICED TOOTH POWDER [2]

Precipitated chalk	1/2 cup
Borax	2 tablespoons
Orrisroot powder	2 tablespoons
Ground cinnamon	1 teaspoon

☞ Combine the ingredients.

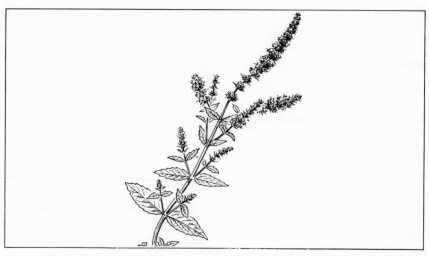

Spearmint is a widely used plant. The oil is a flavoring agent and the dried plant is used in sachets, herbal baths, and facial packs. (Mentha spicata) University of West Virginia.

SWEETENED TOOTH POWDER

Precipitated chalk	1 cup
Camphor	1 teaspoon
Lactose	1 teaspoon
Oil of lime	1/8 teaspoon

☞ Crush the camphor, and mix with the chalk and lactose. Add the oil, and mix well.

VIKING TOOTH POWDER

Precipitated chalk	1 cup
Soap flakes	1/4 cup
Baking soda	1/2 cup
Oil of peppermint	1 teaspoon
Oil of cardamon	1/4 teaspoon

☞ Combine the chalk, soap, and baking soda. Stir in the oils.

VIOLET TOOTH POWDER

Precipitated chalk	2/3 cup
Orrisroot powder	2 tablespoons

| Camphor | 1 1/2 teaspoons |
| Oil of peppermint | 1/8 teaspoon |

☞ Crush the camphor and add to the chalk and the orrisroot. Add the oil.

SWEETENED VIOLET TOOTH POWDER

Precipitated chalk	1 cup
Lactose	3 tablespoons
Orrisroot powder	2 teaspoons
Oil of orange	1/4 teaspoon

☞ Combine all dry ingredients, then add the oil.

TOOTH POWDER WITH STARCH

Precipitated chalk	1 cup
Cornstarch	1 tablespoon
Orrisroot powder	1/4 cup
Oil of lemon	1/4 teaspoon

☞ Combine the dry ingredients, then add the oil.

TOOTHPASTES

CHERRY TOOTHPASTE

Precipitated chalk	1 cup
Orrisroot powder	1/4 cup
Tragacanth	1 teaspoon
Oil of cinnamon	1/4 teaspoon
Cherry juice	2 tablespoons
Glycerin	2 tablespoons
Glucose	2 teaspoons
Water	2 teaspoons

☞ Combine the chalk and the orrisroot. Soften the tragacanth in the water. Combine the oil of cinnamon, cherry juice, glycerin, and glucose with the dry mixture. Add the tragacanth mucilage.

HONEY TOOTHPASTE

Precipitated chalk	3/4 cup
Soap flakes	3 tablespoons
Orrisroot powder	3 tablespoons
Oil of peppermint	1/4 teaspoon
Honey	1/4 cup

☞ Combine the chalk, soap, and orrisroot. Add the honey and the oil, and stir until smooth.

LEMON TOOTHPASTE

Ground lemon peel	3 tablespoons
Ground cinnamon	1 tablespoon
Ground cloves	1 tablespoon
Soap flakes	2 tablespoons
Rose leaves	1 cup
Oil of lemon	1/4 teaspoon
Alcohol, ethyl 50 percent	1/2 cup

☞ Grind the rose leaves and the spices together until fine. Add the soap. Dissolve the oil in the alcohol, and mix into the dry ingredients.

TOOTHPASTE [M]*

Soap flakes	1 cup
Precipitated chalk	1/2 cup
Glycerin	1/2 cup
Oil of peppermint	1/4 teaspoon
Alcohol, ethyl 70 percent	1/2 teaspoon

☞ Combine the soap and the chalk. Add the glycerin, and stir until smooth. Dissolve the oil of peppermint in the alcohol, and add this to the first mixture.

TOOTHPASTE [L]

Precipitated chalk	1 1/3 cups
Soap flakes	3 tablespoons

* Letter designations on this and following pages are for different formulas.

Glycerin	1/4 cup
Oil of peppermint	1/2 teaspoon
Alcohol, ethyl 70 percent	1 teaspoon

☞ Combine the chalk and the soap flakes. Add the glycerin and stir until smooth. Dissolve the oil in the alcohol, and add to the mixture.

TOOTHPASTE [A]

Liquid soap	1 tablespoon
Cornstarch	2 tablespoons
Precipitated chalk	1 cup
Water	1 tablespoon
Glycerin	1 tablespoon
Oil of peppermint	1/4 teaspoon

☞ Combine the cornstarch and the water. Mix until smooth. Add the glycerin, and stir over low heat until a smooth, clear paste is formed. Remove from heat, and stir in the soap, chalk, and oil.

TOOTHPASTE [R]

Sodium carbonate	1 teaspoon
Baking soda	1/4 cup
Glycerin	1 tablespoon
Soap flakes	1 teaspoon
Water	1/2 teaspoon
Oil of peppermint	1/8 teaspoon

☞ Combine the sodium carbonate, baking soda, and soap. Add the glycerin, and stir until smooth. Stir in the water and the oil.

TOOTHPASTE [S]

Precipitated chalk	1 cup
Soap flakes	1/4 cup
Talc	1/4 cup
Granulated sugar	2 tablespoons
Glycerin	1/4 cup
Oil of peppermint	1/2 teaspoon

☞ Combine the chalk, soap, talc, and sugar. Mix in the glycerin and oil to a smooth paste.

TOOTHPASTE [G]

Precipitated chalk	1 cup
Honey	1 tablespoon
Magnesium carbonate	1/4 cup
Soap flakes	1/4 cup
Glycerin	3 tablespoons
Oil of peppermint	1/8 teaspoon

☞ Mix the chalk, honey, soap, and magnesium carbonate together. Add the glycerin, and the oil, and mix until smooth.

TOOTHPASTE [H]

Calcium carbonate	1/2 cup
Kaolin	2 tablespoons
Soap flakes	1 tablespoon
Glycerin	1 1/2 teaspoons
Water	1 tablespoon plus 1 teaspoon
Oil of peppermint	1/4 teaspoon

☞ Combine the calcium carbonate, kaolin, and soap. Add the glycerin, water, and oil, and stir until the paste is smooth.

TOOTHPASTE [B]

Precipitated chalk	1 cup
Talc	2 tablespoons
Orrisroot powder	2 tablespoons
Oil of cinnamon	1/2 teaspoon
Oil of peppermint	1/4 teaspoon
Honey	1/4 cup

☞ Combine the chalk, talc, and orrisroot. Add the honey and oils, and stir until smooth.

TOOTHPASTE [T]

Precipitated chalk	1 1/2 cups
Orrisroot powder	1/4 cup

Glycerin	1/4 cup
Oil of peppermint	1/4 teaspoon
Oil of cinnamon	1/8 teaspoon
Water	1 teaspoon

☞ Combine the chalk and orrisroot. Add the glycerin, water, and oils, and stir until the mixture becomes clear.

TOOTHPASTE [W]

Precipitated chalk	1 cup
Soap flakes	1/4 cup
Orrisroot powder	1 tablespoon
Oil of peppermint	1/4 teaspoon
Alcohol, ethyl 50 percent	1/2 teaspoon
Honey	1/4 cup

☞ Combine the chalk, soap, and orrisroot. Mix with the honey until smooth. Dissolve the oil in the alcohol, and add to the mixture.

TOOTHPASTE [N]

Precipitated chalk	1 cup
Magnesium carbonate	1/4 cup
Orrisroot powder	2 tablespoons
Gelatin	1 teaspoon
Glycerin	2 tablespoons
Water	2 tablespoons

☞ Soften the gelatin in the water. Combine the chalk, magnesium carbonate, and orrisroot. Dissolve the gelatin over low heat, and add the glycerin. Combine with the dry ingredients.

TOOTHPASTE [Q]

Soap flakes	1/2 cup
Talc	1/2 cup
Orrisroot powder	2 tablespoons
Powdered sugar	2 tablespoons
Oil of peppermint	1/4 teaspoon
Water	2 1/2 tablespoons

☞ Combine the soap, talc, orrisroot, and sugar. Add the oil and the water, and mix until smooth.

TOOTHPASTE [E]

Precipitated chalk	2/3 cup
Orrisroot powder	1/4 cup
Liquid soap	1 teaspoon
Borax	1 tablespoon
Honey	1 tablespoon
Glycerin	2 tablespoons

☞ Combine the chalk, borax, and orrisroot. Add the honey, soap, and glycerin.

TOOTHPASTE [K]

Precipitated chalk	2/3 cup
Orrisroot powder	1/4 cup
Soap flakes	1 1/2 tablespoons
Borax	1 1/2 tablespoons
Honey	2 tablespoons
Glycerin	1 1/2 teaspoons

☞ Combine the chalk, orrisroot, soap, and the borax. Add the honey and glycerin, and mix to a smooth paste.

MOUTH WASHES

IMPERIAL WATER [A MOUTH WASH]

Frankincense, benzoin, mastic, gum arabic, cloves, nutmegs, pine-nut kernels, sweet almonds, brandy.

☞ Combine ingredients, using one cup of brandy to one teaspoon of each of the other ingredients. Let steep for three days, then strain.

BERGAMOT MOUTH WASH

Soap flakes	2 tablespoons
Glycerin	1 tablespoon

Water, hot	3/4 cup
Alcohol, ethyl 50 percent	1/4 cup
Oil of bergamot	1/4 teaspoon

☞ Combine the soap and the water. Stir well, then add the glycerin. Dissolve the oil in the alcohol, and add to the water mixture.

CALCUTTA MOUTH WASH

Cream of tartar	1/2 teaspoon
Alcohol, ethyl 50 percent	3/4 cup
Oil of anise	1/8 teaspoon
Oil of cardamon	1/4 teaspoon
Oil of peppermint	1/4 teaspoon
Water	1 3/4 cups

☞ Dissolve the oils in the alcohol. Add the cream of tartar. Stir until it dissolves. Add the water.

CEDAR ISLAND MOUTH WASH

Thymol	1/4 teaspoon
Alcohol, ethyl 70 percent	1/4 cup
Glycerin	1/4 cup
Soap flakes	1 teaspoon
Oil of cedarwood	1/4 teaspoon
Oil of peppermint	1/8 teaspoon
Water, hot	1 1/2 cups

☞ Dissolve the soap flakes in the water. Dissolve the oils and the thymol in the alcohol. Combine the water and alcohol mixtures, and stir in the glycerin.

CINNAMON MOUTH WASH

Star anise	1/2 teaspoon
Ground cloves	1/4 teaspoon
Ground cinnamon	1/4 teaspoon
Alcohol, ethyl 60 percent	1/2 cup
Water	1 1/2 cups
Oil of orange	1/4 teaspoon
Oil of cinnamon	1/8 teaspoon

☞ Add the spices to the alcohol. Let set for three days, then strain. Add the oils and the water.

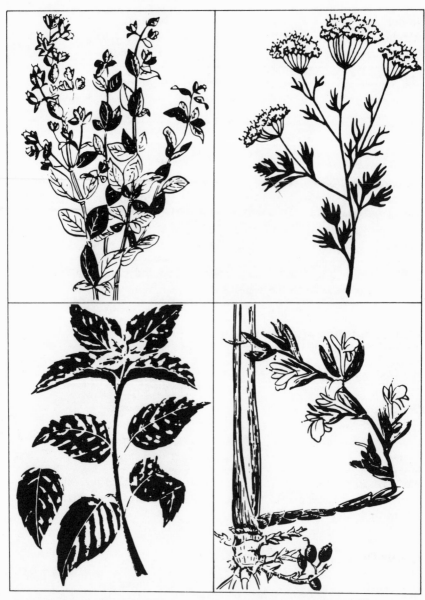

Upper left, marjoram (Majorana hortensis); **upper right, anise** (Pimpinella anisum); **lower left, basil** (Ocimum basilicum); **lower right, cardamon** (Elettaria cardamomum). American Spice Trade Association.

CITRON MOUTH WASH

Oil of citron	1/8 teaspoon
Thymol	1/2 teaspoon
Menthol	1/4 teaspoon
Tincture of eucalyptus	2 tablespoons
Water	2 cups

☞ Dissolve the thymol and the menthol in the tincture of eucalyptus. Add the oil and the water.

CLOVE MOUTH WASH

Tincture of cloves	1 teaspoon
Oil of cloves	1/8 teaspoon
Borax	1/2 teaspoon
Water	2 cups

☞ Dissolve the borax in the water. Add the tincture and the oil.

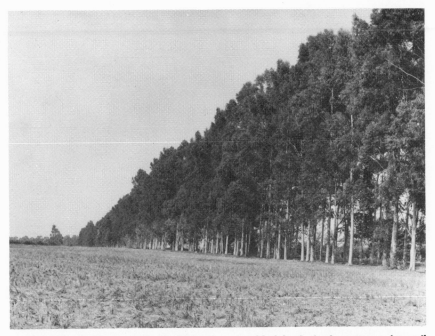

The stately eucalyptus, with its distinctive shredded bark, is the source of an oil used as a flavoring in toothpaste and mouth washes. The trees are found in California, Australia, Israel, and Brazil. (Eucalyptus spp.) Arnold Krochmal.

CORIANDER MOUTH WASH

Oil of coriander	1/4 teaspoon
Tincture of myrrh	1 teaspoon
Water	1 1/2 cups
Alcohol, ethyl 60 percent	1/4 cup

☞ Combine the ingredients.

LEMON MOUTH WASH

Alcohol, ethyl 70 percent	1/2 cup
Water	2 cups
Oil of lemon	1 teaspoon
Oil of cloves	1/8 teaspoon

☞ Dissolve the oils in the alcohol. Add the water.

LIME MOUTH WASH

Alcohol, ethyl 60 percent	1/4 cup
Soap flakes	1/4 teaspoon
Water, hot	1 cup
Oil of lime	1/4 teaspoon

☞ Dissolve the soap in the water. Dissolve the oil in the alcohol, and add to the water mixture.

DOUBLE MINT MOUTH WASH

Benzoic acid	1/8 teaspoon
Thymol	1/8 teaspoon
Tincture of cedarwood	1/2 teaspoon
Oil of peppermint	5 drops
Oil of spearmint	5 drops
Alcohol, ethyl 50 percent	1/2 cup

☞ Dissolve the oils, benzoic acid, and thymol in the alcohol. Add the tincture.

ORANGE MOUTH WASH

Water	2 cups
Menthol	1/4 teaspoon
Oil of eucalyptus	1/8 teaspoon
Oil of orange	1/4 teaspoon
Alcohol, ethyl 70 percent	1/2 cup

☞ Dissolve the menthol and the oils in the alcohol. Add the water.

PEPPERMINT MOUTH WASH

Soap flakes	1/2 teaspoon
Alcohol, ethyl 55 percent	1/4 cup
Water, hot	1 cup
Glycerin	1/4 cup
Oil of cloves	1/8 teaspoon
Oil of peppermint	1/4 teaspoon
Tincture of vanilla	1 tablespoon

☞ Dissolve the soap in the water. Dissolve the oils in the alcohol, and add to the water mixture. Add the glycerin and the tincture of vanilla.

SAGE MOUTH WASH

Alcohol, ethyl 60 percent	1/2 cup
Oil of orange	1/4 teaspoon
Oil of sage	1/8 teaspoon
Water	2 cups

☞ Dissolve the oils in the alcohol. Add the water.

SPEARMINT MOUTH WASH

Alcohol, ethyl 60 percent	1/2 cup plus 2 tablespoons
Tincture of cedarwood	2 tablespoons
Oil of spearmint	1/4 teaspoon
Water	1 1/2 cups

☞ Dissolve the oil in the alcohol. Add the tincture of cedarwood and water.

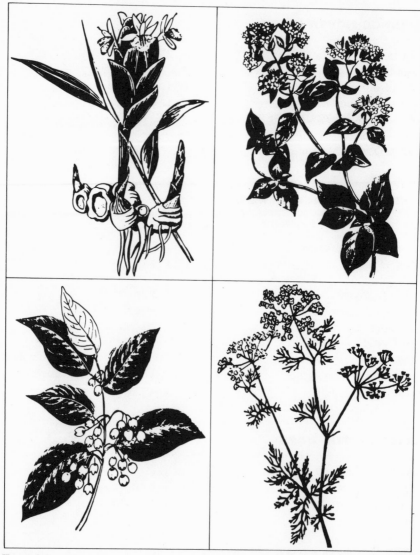

Upper left, ginger (Zingiber officinale); **upper right, oregano** (Origanum vulgare); **lower left, nutmeg** (Myristica fragrans); **lower right, caraway** (Carum carvi). American Spice Trade Association.

KITCHEN SPICE MOUTH WASH

Ground cinnamon	1 teaspoon
Ground cloves	1 teaspoon
Ground allspice	1/4 teaspoon
Aniseed	1 tablespoon
Alcohol, ethyl 65 percent	1/2 cup

| Oil of peppermint | 1/2 teaspoon |
| Water | 1 3/4 cups |

☞ Let the spices set in the alcohol for a week. Strain, and add the oil and the water.

SPICED MINT MOUTH WASH

Oil of spearmint	1/8 teaspoon
Oil of cloves	1/8 teaspoon
Oil of cinnamon	1/8 teaspoon
Water	1 cup
Alcohol, ethyl 60 percent	1/4 cup

☞ Dissolve the oils in the alcohol. Add the water.

FLORAL SPICE MOUTH WASH

Cream of tartar	1/2 teaspoon
Orange-flower water	1/4 cup
Ground cinnamon	1/4 teaspoon
Ground ginger	1/4 teaspoon
Aniseed	1/2 teaspoon
Alcohol, ethyl 50 percent	1/2 cup
Water	1 1/2 cups

☞ Combine the cinnamon, ginger, aniseed, and alcohol. Let set for a day. Add the cream of tartar, and orange-flower water. Let set for a day. Add the water.

SPICE-FLAVORED MOUTH WASH

Angelica root powder	2 teaspoons
Aniseed	2 teaspoons
Ground cinnamon	1/2 teaspoon
Ground allspice	1/8 teaspoon
Alcohol, ethyl 50 percent	1/2 cup
Oil of peppermint	1/4 teaspoon
Water	1 1/2 cups

☞ Let the spices set in the alcohol for a week. Strain, then add the oil and water.

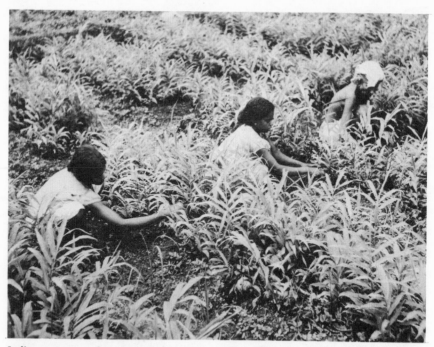

Indian women cultivating ginger plants. The spice comes from a tuberous root, now grown in the West Indies as well as India, Africa, and parts of the Far East. The roots are carefully dried and most often peeled before being shipped to this country. (Zingiber officinale) American Spice Trade Association.

SPICY MOUTH WASH

Ground cinnamon	2 teaspoons
Ground cloves	1/4 teaspoon
Ground ginger	1/4 teaspoon
Oil of cinnamon	1/4 teaspoon
Alcohol, ethyl 70 percent	1/3 cup
Water	1 1/2 cups

☞ Let the spices set in the alcohol for a week. Strain, then add the oil and the water.

TASMANIAN MOUTH WASH

Soap flakes	1/4 cup
Thymol	1/4 teaspoon
Glycerin	1 tablespoon

Alcohol, ethyl 70 percent	1/4 cup
Water, hot	1 cup
Oil of eucalyptus	1/8 teaspoon
Oil of orange	1/4 teaspoon

☞ Dissolve the soap in the water. Add the glycerin. Dissolve the thymol and the oils in the alcohol, then add to the water mixture.

THYMOL MOUTH WASH

Oil of spearmint	1/8 teaspoon
Tincture of cedarwood	2 tablespoons
Alcohol, ethyl 50 percent	1 1/2 cups
Water	1 cup
Thymol	1/4 teaspoon

☞ Dissolve the thymol and oil in the alcohol. Add the water and tincture of cedarwood.

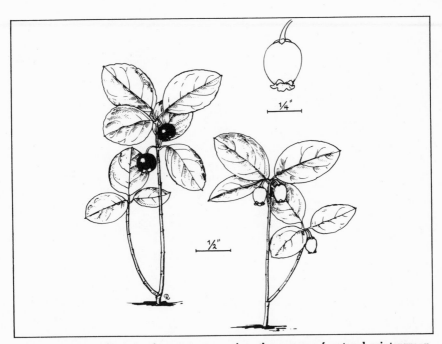

Wintergreen is a low-growing evergreen vine, the source of natural wintergreen. The plant has bright red berries. (Gaultheria procumbens) U.S. Forest Service.

WINTERGREEN-ROSE MOUTH WASH

Rosewater	1 tablespoon
Oil of wintergreen	1/2 teaspoon
Water	2 cups
Alcohol, ethyl 60 percent	1/2 cup

☞ Dissolve the oil in the alcohol. Add the rosewater and the water.

MOUTH WASH CONCENTRATE

Thymol	1/8 teaspoon
Menthol	1/8 teaspoon
Oil of eucalyptus	1/8 teaspoon
Tincture of myrrh	1 teaspoon
Alcohol, ethyl 60 percent	1/4 cup
Water	1 cup

☞ Dissolve the thymol, menthol, and oil of eucalyptus in the alcohol. Add the tincture of myrrh and the water. For use, dilute in two or three times as much water.

DESCRIPTIONS
OF NATURAL MATERIALS
USED IN FORMULAS

Agar-Agar: Agar-agar is an extract of red algae, which are collected in the summer and fall, and then dried. The manufacture of the agar begins in cold weather and usually runs from November to February. After drying, it is washed, cooked with hot water to extract the gelatin, cooled, frozen, and crushed; when dried, the flakes are ready for use. In Japan, algae are encouraged to grow on poles sunk into the water along the seacoast; they can then be collected from the poles. (*Gelidium cartilagineum*, Rhodophyllaceae)

Allspice: See PIMENTA.

Almond, Bitter: Volatile oil is obtained from the dried ripe kernels of a variety of almond trees. (*Amygdalus communis* var. *amara*)

Almond, Sweet: Same as above, but it comes from a different variety of almond. (*Amygdalus communis*)

Ambrette: A muskmallow plant whose seeds are the source of an oil that has an odor resembling musk. (*Hibiscus abelmoschus*)

Angelica Root: A root product from any one of several angelicas. (*Angelica* spp.)

Anise, Oil of: Anise is cultivated in many localities for its seeds, but is grown principally in the Soviet Union. (*Pimpinella anisum*)

Anise, Star: A small tree, producing fruit an inch in diameter, which is native to China, Korea, and Japan and is now found in the Southeastern United States. (*Illicium anisatum*)

Arnica Flowers: Arnica is a perennial plant whose flower heads are collected when they are open. European arnica comes mostly from Germany, Belgium, Yugoslavia, France, and Italy. American arnica comes from the Rocky Mountain states, especially Montana, Wyoming, and the Dakotas. (*Arnica* spp.)

Balsam, Balm of Gilead, Mecca Myrrh: A series of trees that grow in the Arabian peninsula near Medina and Mecca, and yield a gummy substance. Incisions are made in the bark of the tree to induce the flow of the resin, which is aged in earthenware pots and then distilled to get the oil. (Balm of Gilead: *Commiphora opobalsam*)

Balsam of Peru, or Peru Balsam: A tree of Central America, principally El Salvador, on whose trunk a gumlike substance is found around scars and wounds. (*Myroxylon balsamum*)

Barberry: The bark of this plant is used in hair preparations as a conditioner and dye. (*Berberis vulgaris*)

Bay Oil: Sweet bay oil comes from seeds of a tree of the Mediterranean area. (*Laurus nobilis*) The west Indian bay tree, introduced to the Caribbean islands of Barbados, Jamaica, and Antigua from the East Indies, is the source of bay oil distilled from its leaves and fruits. (*Myrcia acris* or *Pimenta acris*)

Bay Rum: Bay rum is produced by distilling the leaves of the bay tree in crude rum or by dissolving the bay oil in alcohol. (*Myrcia acris* or *Pimenta acris*)

Benzoin, Tincture of (Storax, Styrax): Benzoin is collected from trees much as pine resin is. The trees grow principally in Thailand, Java, and Borneo. (*Styrax benzoin*)

Bergamot, Oil of: The oil, manufactured from the rind of the lemon-shaped fruits of a citrus tree, is imported from Sicily. (*Citrus bergamia*)

Black Hellebore: A perennial plant native to the mountainous regions of southern Europe. It is called Christmas rose because it blooms in winter. (*Helleborus niger*)

Broad Bean: This large, flat bean is sold canned or dried. (*Vicia faba*)

Broom: A native European shrub, also found in the United States, from which the flowers are collected. (*Sarothamnus scoparius*)

Calamus (Sweet Flag): The roots of this plant, growing in sweet water, are aromatic and when dried are used in sachets. Calamus oil is used in perfumes. (*Acorus calamus*)

Camphor: The product of a tree native to China and Japan. Camphor sold as "synthetic" is the result of a method of pushing the yields of young trees. (*Cinnamomum camphora*)

Caraway: The aromatic seeds of this plant, grown in U.S. gardens, are used for an oil obtained by distillation. It is a very old plant, and seeds have been found in ancient Swiss lake dwellings. (*Carum carvi*)

Cardamon: Cardamon seeds and seed oil are used in colognes. The plant is grown in gardens in the United States. (*Elettaria cardamonum*)

Carob (St. John's Bread): This Mediterranean tree produces beans in a large pod, from which an alcohol is made. The pod is also a source of a vegetable gum often used instead of tragacanth, especially in creams. (*Ceratonia siliqua*)

Carthamus: A red pigment derived from safflower flowers. (*Carthamus tinctorius*)

Cassie: A number of species of trees and shrubs whose bark produces a gum resembling gum arabic. Extracts of the flowers produce a perfume concentrate and an oil. (*Acacia spp.*) In the United

States, European black currant has been used to produce a similar oil. (*Ribes nigrum*)

Castor Oil: The beans of a tropical shrub or tree, castor oil plant, are pressed to yield this oil. (*Ricinus communis*)

Cedarwood Oil: Red cedar is the source of this oil, which is used in perfumes, soap, and shaving preparations. (*Juniperus virginiana*)

Chamomile: This European plant produces an oil used in perfumes and shampoos. The flowers make a fine sachet. (*Matricaria chamomilla*) Roman, or English, chamomile resembles true chamomile. (*Anthemis nobilis*)

Cinchona Bark: The bark from a number of South American trees has been used as a source of quinine for treatment of malaria, and is used as a preservative in perfumery. Some of the trees are cultivated in Java and Indonesia. (*Cinchona* spp.)

Citronella: Several related tropical grasses from Asia are the source of oil of citronella, used in colognes and soaps. (*Cymbopogon nardus*)

Citron Oil: This oil is produced from the peel of the fruit of citron, probably the only orange known in ancient Rome. (*Citrus medica*)

Cloves: Cloves are the dried flower buds of a tropical tree that grows in Sumatra, Zanzibar, and the West Indies. They also yield an aromatic oil. (*Eugenia caryophyllata*)

Cocoa Butter: This extract from the cocoa bean, a seed of the cocoa tree, is used in creams and suntan lotions. (*Theobroma cacao*)

Coconut Oil: A product of the fruit of the coconut palm, coconut oil is used in soaps, cosmetics, shampoos, shaving creams, and face creams. (*Cocos nucifera*)

Comfrey Roots: The roots of the comfrey plant, which is found in the United States, are used as a skin softener and astringent. (*Symphytum officinale*)

Coriander: The spicy fruits are used to flavor foods and gin; and the oil derived from coriander seeds is used in perfumes and soaps. (*Coriandrum sativum*)

Deerstongue: This plant is harvested in our Southeastern states, mainly Florida and Georgia; its leaves smell and taste like vanilla. (*Trilisa odoratissima*)

Elder Flower: The American elder, a shrub or tree, produces the flowers used to make elder-flower water. (*Sambucus canadensis*) The European tree is used for the same purpose, and in Europe the flowers are also used as a mouth-wash material. (*Sambucus nigra*)

Eucalyptus: Oil of eucalyptus comes from the leaves of the Australian eucalyptus tree. Eucalyptol is what gives the oil the qualities desired in perfumes. (*Eucalyptus globulus*)

Fennel: The dried fruit of this lacy plant, as well as its roots, are the sources of oil of fennel. (*Foeniculum vulgare*)

Frankincense: This is the gum exuded by a small tree of the Middle East. It is used in perfumes, soaps, and sachets. (*Boswellia carteri*)

Geranium: Oil of geranium is distilled from leaves of several related plants, all with sweet-smelling foliage. (*Pelargonium odoratissimum* and others)

Ginger: This popular spice comes from the roots of the tropical ginger plant, as does a pungent oil. Ginger is also used in cosmetics for an Oriental touch. (*Zingiber officinale*)

Glucose: Known as dextrose and grape sugar, glucose is found in various fruits and honey.

Gum Acacia: Gum acacia and gum arabic are collected from the stem and branches of the acacia, a tree or shrub. (*Acacia senegal* and others)

Gum Karaya: A gum similar to tragacanth. (*Sterculia urens*)

Henna: An Egyptian shrub that is the source of a bright brown dye, usually for the hair but men in the Near East and Central Asia use it around their eyes and sometimes on the palms of the hands. (*Lawsonia alba*)

Hops: The dried ripe cones of the female flowers of hop, a cultivated vine. The essential oil from these cones is used in perfume. (*Humulus lupulus*)

Irish Moss: This red alga, found in the North Atlantic, is used in lotions, creams, hair preparations, toothpastes, and shaving creams. (*Chondrus crispus*)

Jasmine: Several species of jasmine yield an essential oil used in perfumery. (*Jasminum*)

Laurel: Various species of laurel shrubs contain an oil used in perfumery. (*Laurus* spp.)

Lavender: The flowering tops of lavender plants are distilled to produce an oil for perfumes. The dried flowers have long been used in sachets and for toilet vinegars. (*Lavandula* spp.)

Lemon: This popular and common citrus fruit is the source of oil of lemon, used in perfumes; the seeds are the source of lemon seed oil, used in soap. (*Citrus limon*)

Lemon Grass: This designates a group of tropical grasses yielding an oil with a strong odor of lemon or of violets. (*Cymbopogon* spp.)

Licorice: The well-known licorice flavoring comes from the roots of several related plants. Licorice-root water is made by simply soaking the roots in water. (*Glycyrrhiza* spp.)

Lilac: The highly scented flowers are a frequent component of sachets. (*Syringa vulgaris*)

Lime, Oil of: Oil of lime is pressed from the peel of this green or yellow citrus fruit. (*Citrus aurantifolia*)

Linden Flowers: The flowers are collected from the linden shrub and used as an astringent in washes, facial masks, and bath preparations. (*Tilia cordata*)

Linette: An oil is obtained from the thick peel of the citrus fruit, and used in perfumery. The "etrog" of the Bible, used by Jews during the Feast of the Tabernacle, is a relative. (*Citrus medica*)

Linseed: The seeds of the flax plant, also called flaxseeds, are the source of linseed oil. In addition to its many practical applications, it is used to make mucilages. (*Linum usitatissimum*)

Locust Bean Gum: See CAROB.

Lycopodium: This clubmoss produces spores used in powders and sachets. (*Lycopodium clavatum*)

Mace: The plant that gives us the seed known as nutmeg also gives us mace. Mace is the outer covering of the seed. (*Myristica fragrans*)

Marjoram: A culinary herb which is the source of an essential oil. (*Majorana hortensis*)

Mastic Gum: This resinous substance is exuded from the bark of the mastic tree. In parts of Asia it is chewed to clean the teeth and make the breath pleasant. (*Pistacia lentiscus*)

Melissa: Oil of melissa, or oil of balm, is sometimes a mixture of oil of citronella and oil of lemon because so little oil is produced from the melissa plant itself. (*Melissa officinalis*)

Menthol: An alcohol-like material obtained from oil of the peppermint plant. Our menthol generally comes from Japan. (*Mentha piperita*)

Mignonette, Oil of: The oil is obtained from the garden mignonette, widely cultivated in France. (*Reseda odorata*)

Milk Sugar—Lactose: A sugar found in milk.

Mint: A highly aromatic group of plants including spearmint and peppermint. The essential oil is much used in dentrifices, mouth washes, and sachets. (*Mentha piperita* and *Mentha spicata*)

Myrrh: A gum obtained from wounds made in the trunk of a group of trees and shrubs of Africa and India. Tincture of myrrh is the powdered gum in alcohol. (*Commiphora* spp.)

Narcissus: The flowers are the source of an oil much used in perfumes of mixed floral scents and whenever an exotic Oriental effect is desired. (*Narcissus* spp.)

Neroli: An oil, distilled from the flower of the sour orange tree, that is frequently used in perfumes. (*Citrus aurantium*)

Nettle: This usually troublesome plant with its stinging hairs, is used for hair washes; the seeds are used for hair conditioners. (*Urtica dioica*)

Orange, Oil of: The fresh peel of bitter orange yields a bitter oil. (*Citrus aurantium*)

Orrisroot: The dried powdered root of the Florentine iris is used in tooth powder, dusting powders, and sachets. The oil from the root is used in violet perfumes. (*Iris florentina*). Closely related is the German iris. (*Iris germanica*)

Patchouly: A shrubby East Indian mint plant whose leaves yield a fragrant oil used in perfume and soap. The dried leaves may be scattered over stored clothes to add a pleasant scent. (*Pogostemon* spp.)

Pimenta: An oil produced from the fruit and leaves of allspice grown in Jamaica. (*Pimenta officinalis*)

Pine Needle Oil: A distillation from the needles of Scotch pine. (*Pinus sylvestris*)

Pinus Pumilio: This oil, also called dwarf pine needle oil, is used widely in toiletries requiring a pine scent. (*Pinus pumilio*)

Privet: This is a common shrub often used to form a hedge. In medieval England the leaves were a part of complexion washes, shampoos, and other cosmetics. (*Ligustrum vulgare*)

Psyllium Seed: The seeds of this plant, belonging to the plantain family are used in hair-setting compounds because they produce a thick mucilage. (*Plantago psyllium*)

Quince Seed: From the seeds of the quince fruit comes a mucilage used in cold creams, hair lotions, and wavesets. In China, the fruits of a related species are used to provide a pleasing scent in closets and other rooms. (*Cydonia sinensis*)

Reseda: See MIGNONETTE.

Rhatany: The powdered root of this plant, native to South America, is a light tan or rust color and has been used in tooth powders. (*Krameria triandra*)

Rhodium: Oil of rhodium, sometimes called rosewood oil, is extracted from the roots of this plant. Both the oil and the plant itself are used in perfumery and soap production. (*Convolvulus scoparius* and *Convolvulus floridus*)

Rose Oil: This oil is obtained by the distillation of rose petals. (*Rosa* spp.)

Rose Geranium Oil: See GERANIUM.

Rosewater, Stronger: After rose oil has been removed from distilled rose flowers, the remaining liquid is called stronger rosewater. Adding an equal volume of distilled water produces rosewater. (*Rosa* spp.)

Rosemary, Oil of: This oil is distilled from the leaves and flowers of an aromatic evergreen plant, well known as a cooking herb. The dried plant and the oil are used in colognes, mouth washes, and perfumes. (*Rosmarinus officinalis*)

Rue: A culinary herb, rue is the source of an essential oil used in perfumery. (*Ruta* spp.)

Sage: The garden sage plant, source of the much-used seasoning herb associated with turkey, also produces an oil used in perfumes, mouth washes, and sachets. (*Salvia officinalis*)

Sandalwood: Oil and wood are produced by this tropical tree of India and Malaya. The wood is used as a sachet, and the oil is used in perfumery (*Santalum album*). Red sandalwood, also called sandalwood, does not produce oil, but the wood is highly aromatic and used in sachets. (*Adenanthera pavonina* L.)

Sassafras: This common eastern tree is highly aromatic. Crushing a leave in your hand will release an attractive scent. The bark has been used for tea and is still used in Appalachia. An oil from the bark has been used for flavoring and as an antiseptic. (*Sassafras albidum*)

Sesame Seed: The seeds of the sesame plant are used not only in cooking but in hair preparations. An oil is also extracted from them. (*Sesamum indicum*)

Storax: This gummy material collected from a fragrant tree, found in Asia Minor and related to witch hazel, is used in soaps and perfumes. (*Liquidambar orientalis*) In America, storax is produced by our familiar sweet gum tree. (*Liquidambar styraciflua*)

Strawberry: Both the berries and the foliage are used as astringents in cosmetics, and an essential oil of the plant is used in soap, creams, shampoos, bath preparations, and perfumery. (*Fragaria virginiana*)

Tar Oil: The pine tar obtained by distilling the wood of pine trees is the source of this oil.

Terpineol: The turpentine that comes from pine trees produces this alcohol with a lilac odor, widely used in perfumes. (*Pinus palustris*)

Thuja Oil: From the needles of arborvitae, a native American evergreen tree, comes an oil used in perfumes and after-shave lotions. (*Thuja occidentalis*)

Thyme Oil: This oil is distilled from the entire thyme plant, a well-known cooking herb. (*Thymus vulgaris*)

Tolu Balsam: A very sticky, thick exudation is collected from balsam-of-Tolu trees in tropical South America, just as maple-tree sap is collected for syrup. The balsam is used as a fixative and to create an Oriental type of perfume. (*Myroxylon balsamum*)

Tonka: A tree whose fruit is a bean with a strong vanilla odor, much used in perfumery. (*Dipteryx odorata*)

Tragacanth: A gummy discharge from injuries on the stems of certain East European and Asiatic plants. It is used in wavesets, lotions, creams, and toothpastes. (*Astragalus gummifer*)

Tuberose Oil: The sweet-smelling flowers of this bulbous plant produce an oil used in quality perfumes. (*Polianthes tuberosa*)

Turpentine Oil: This oil is distilled from pine-tree resin. (*Pinus palustris*)

Vanilla: A lovely American climbing orchid produces vanilla beans in a pod, from which oil of vanilla and tincture of vanilla are made. These are widely used in cosmetic preparations, as well as in cooking. (*Vanilla planifolia*)

Verbena: Verbena, highly esteemed in Egypt and Greece, is the source of an essential oil with a light, delicate lemon aroma, used in perfumery, creams, and colognes. (*Lippia citriodora* and others)

Vetiver: The roots of this Asiatic grass are used in sachets. An essential oil from the roots is used in soaps, creams, and perfumery. (*Vetiveria zizanoides*)

Wintergreen: Partridgeberry, a low-growing, attractive forest plant with shiny leaves and bright red fruit, yields oil of wintergreen for toothpastes, mouth washes, and hair preparations. (*Gaultheria procumbens*)

Witch Hazel: The bark and leaves of this tree, long used by the Indians, are the source of our familiar witch hazel. This highly astringent distilled product is much used in face lotions, friction lotions, and after-shave preparations. (*Hamamelis virginiana*)

NATURAL MINERALS

Alum: May be obtained from one of several naturally occurring minerals, among which are bauxite, cryolite, and alum stone. Certain soils are also sources of alum. (*Potassium alum* and *Ammonium alum*)

Ammonia: A colorless gas made of nitrogen and hydrogen. Ammonia and its compounds are found naturally in air, water, plants, and animal urine, as well as deposits of guano. Ammonia is produced mainly as a result of the burning of coal and as a by-product in certain industries. Some is made by combining nitrogen and hydrogen. *Ammonia water* is a solution of the gas in water. (NH_3)

Benzoic Acid: Used as a preservative, it is isolated from benzoin by heating. (See BENZOIN.)

Borax: A compound found naturally in the western United States. It is used as a preservative and cleanser. ($Na_2B_4O_7$)

Boric Acid: A compound found in both saltwater and mineral springs, in natural deposits in South America, and in bodies of water near volcanoes. Used in creams and lotions as a preservative. (H_3BO_3)

Calcium Carbonate: Found in seashells (such as oyster shells), teeth, bones, and in deposits of marble, chalk, and limestone. ($CaCO_3$)

Chalk: Venetian or French chalk is made of chalk finely ground and heated, then mixed with small amounts of essential oils. Chalk is used in toothpastes and tooth powders, rouges, and creams.

Epsom Salts: Found in mineral springs, seawater, and caves; is used in bath preparations. (*Magnesium sulfate*, Mg SO_47H_2O)

Fuller's Earth: A very absorbent mixture of silica and clay used in tooth powders and bath preparations.

Kaolin (China Clay): A clay material of high purity found in the United States and Europe. It is used in tooth powders, bath powders, and creams.

Magnesium Carbonate: Occurs in nature as a mineral and is found in seawater. It is used in body powders, toothpastes, rouge, and perfumes. (MgO)

Mineral Oil: A by-product of petroleum refining, also known as liquid petrolatum. It is used in cold creams, bath preparations, and cleansing creams.

Petroleum Jelly: A semisolid by-product of petroleum refining used in cold creams, lotions, cuticle softeners, and a wide range of other cosmetics.

Potassium Carbonate (Potash): Has been obtained from sugar beet molasses, sheep's wool and in the past from wood ashes. (K_2CO_3)

Sulfur: An element found in volcanic areas and in Sicily, Texas, Louisiana, and Mexico. It is sometimes used in ointments. (S)

Talc: A soft mineral used in powders of all sorts and in toothpastes and tooth powders. (*Magnesium silicate*)

SOAPS

Castile Soap: A soap made from olive oil and soda.

Green Soap: Made from linseed oil and potash, or any vegetable oil other than coconut oil.

Green Soap, Tincture of: Made by adding alcohol and lavender oil to green soap.

INSECT AND ANIMAL MATERIALS

Beeswax: A by-product of honey production, also called white wax.

Carmine: A reddish dye made from the body of the female scale insect *cochineal*. It is used as coloring matter in a wide range of cosmetics. (*Coccos cacti*)

Glycerin: A liquid obtained from several sources. It has been made from sugar; from petroleum as a by-product of fermentation; and from soap as a by-product. It is used as a skin softener in creams and lotions, shaving creams, and toothpastes.

Lanolin: A skin-softening fatty material obtained from sheeps' wool. It is used in cold creams, shaving creams, lotions, and cleansing creams.

Stearic Acid: A waxlike, fatty substance obtained from animal and vegetable fats.

ESSENTIAL OILS

The list of plants used to produce essential oils is a long one. In this book those mentioned most frequently are thyme, the source of thymol; mint from spearmint or peppermint; lavender; and bay. The appendix includes a table showing some of the more important sources of these precious oils.

Rose oil is one of the most desired for perfumes and perhaps the most expensive, selling for as much as $100 an ounce when bought in small quantities. The Soviet Union is probably the world's largest producer of this really precious oil, accounting for over 60 percent of world production. An experiment station in the Crimea produces between 1,700 and 1,800 pounds of rose oil per year.

The Soviets have also developed a new variety of rose geranium that produces 150 percent more oil than any standard source as well as a lavender producing 20 to 30 percent more oil than older varieties.

The United States is the world's largest producer of mint oils, used both as oils (in chewing gum and toothpastes, for example) and as a source of menthol production. Brazil produces a low quality of mint oil known as corn oil, and mainland China produces small quantities of mint oil.

Mint production in the United States has been moving westward from its original home in the New England states to New York, Ohio, and Michigan, and finally to its present home in the Northwest, particularly Oregon and Washington. Spearmint production is concentrated in the Yakima Valley of Washington State, while peppermint is widely grown in the Yakima Valley and Columbia Basin of Washington, and the Willamette Valley and Madras Plateau of Oregon.

Florida is producing increasing amounts of excellent citrus oils: orange, lemon, lime, and grapefruit. I have used these in some of the formulas and have found them lovely—gentle, clean, and clearly identifiable.

OIL YIELDS
PER HUNDRED POUNDS
OF SELECTED PLANTS

Almonds	7 ozs.	Marjoram	1 lb.
Aniseed	1 3/4–3 lbs.	Myrtle	4 1/2 ozs.
Balm, or melissa	1 2/3–2 1/2 ozs.	Nutmeg	9–11 lbs.
Calamus root	12–16 ozs.	Orange peel	10 ozs.
Caraway seed	4 lbs.	Patchouly	1 1/2 lbs.
Cassia	12 ozs.	Peppermint	12–16 ozs.
Castor bean	20–50 lbs.	Rhodium	2 1/3–3 1/2 ozs.
Cedarwood	13 ozs.	Rose blooms	1/8–1/4 oz.
Cinnamon	12 ozs.	Rose geranium leaves	1 3/4 ozs.
Cloves	15–18 lbs.	Sandalwood	1 1/2 lbs.
Hops	1/4–1 oz.	Thyme	5–7 1/2 ozs.
Lavender	2 lbs.	Vetiver	13 ozs.
Mace	9 lbs.	Violet	1/8 oz.

ANIMAL PRODUCTS

A number of animal by-products have been used in the perfumery and cosmetic trade. I have deliberately omitted any reference formulas using such products because of the cruelty to, and possible extinction of, the animals involved. Following is a list of the by-products, with explanations of the means used to collect each one.

Castor: The source was the beaver of either sex. A white, creamy liquid found in the sacs in the animal's body between its hind legs was used as a fixative in perfumes. The only way to get the material was to kill the animal. In the past most castor came from Canada and the Soviet Union.

Civet: This secretion from the civet cat is similar to castor and was used in much the same way. The live animal was forced to secrete civet by enclosing it in a cage so narrow that it could not turn around and by irritating it until it became angry. The material discharged was then removed from the cat by means of a spatula. The animals were not killed but continuously tormented.

Musk: This secretion, similar to castor and civet and used for the same purposes, is produced by male musk deer. Unhappily, in the past musk-seekers made no distinction between male and female deer. Thus about half of the animals killed for musk failed to produce any. The average yield of musk per deer is about two ounces. Musklike oils are also produced by muskrats as well as by some plants, including the seed of hibiscus and a Near Eastern plant, sumbul (*Ferula sumbul*). Sumbul is used as a perfume and an incense. Synthetic musk is available.

Whale Products: The importation of any whale products into the United States has been banned, and so their use here is not a problem. In the past, two products were much in demand: [1] **Ambergris.** This waxlike material from the whale's intestines was sometimes found floating in the sea and occasionally on beaches. It was hailed with joy by the crews of whalers because of its very high value as a fixative in the perfume industry. [2] **Spermaceti.** This solid, waxlike substance was found in the head of the sperm whale and some kinds of dolphins. It was used in candles as well as in ointments and creams.

SOME SOURCES
OF MATERIALS

Bekal Products Company
Cruz-Bustillo, Hari
565 Southwest 22nd Street
Miami, Florida 33135

Dried flowers and herbs

Boericke and Tafel
1011 Arch Street
Philadelphia, Pennsylvania 19107

Tinctures and extracts

Capriland Herb Farm
Coventry, Connecticut 06238

Oils, gums, resins, barks, potpourri materials

Hortica Garden
P.O. Box 308
Placerville, California 95767

Dried flowers

Indiana Botanic Gardens
P.O. Box 5
Hammond, Indiana 46325

Flowers, gums, resins, tinctures, extracts, oils, dry herbs

Nature's Herb Company
381 Ellis Street
San Francisco, California 94102

Oils, extracts, tinctures, dry herbs and flowers

The Oriental Store of Raleigh
3121 North Boulevard
King's Plaza Shopping Center
Raleigh, North Carolina 27604

Flours of lentil, chick-pea, rice,
spices, agar-agar, coconut oil

Shuttle Hill Herb Shop
2368 Delaware Avenue
Delmar, New York 12054

Herbs and spices

Topanga Sun Products
133 South Topanga Canyon Blvd.
Topanga, California 90290

Natural oils of blueberry,
cucumber, cinnamon, lemon,
lemon-lime, patchouly,
patchouly-mint, raspberry,
tangerine, vanilla, cherry
bergamot

DEFINITIONS

I have noted some confusion in writings on perfumery regarding certain materials. These definitions may be of help to the beginning cosmetics craftsman.

Extract—Any material which has been extracted from plant materials by a range of methods. Extract of witch hazel and extract of vanilla are two familiar examples. The plant material is steeped in a suitable liquid. If the liquid is alcohol the resulting extract may be called:

Essence, spirit, otto, or *attar*—These are usually an essential oil (volatile oil) dissolved in alcohol.

PREPARING ALCOHOL OF VARYING STRENGTHS

TO GET	ADD TO 1 CUP OF 70% ALCOHOL
65%	3 tablespoons water
60%	4 tablespoons water
55%	5 tablespoons water
50%	6 tablespoons water

TO GET	ADD TO 1 CUP OF 95% ALCOHOL
90%	1 tablespoon water
85%	2 tablespoons water
80%	3 tablespoons water
75%	5 tablespoons water
70%	7 tablespoons water
65%	1/2 cup of water
60%	1/2 cup + 1 tablespoon water
55%	1/2 cup + 3 tablespoons water
50%	3/4 cup water

SOME ASTRINGENT PLANTS

NAME	PART USED	BOTANICAL NAME
Acacia	Green fruits	*Acacia*
Ash	Bark	*Fraxinus*
Bayberry	Bark, root, root bark	*Myrica*
Boneset	Root, foliage	*Eupatorium*
Broom-rape	Plant	*Orobanche*
Chinaberry	Leaves	*Melia*
Chinquapin	Bark	*Castanea*
Dock	Root	*Rumex*
Geranium	Leaves, entire plant	*Geranium*
Goldenrod	Plant	*Solidago*
Hickory	Leaves	*Carya*
Huckleberry	Fruits	*Vaccinium*
Knotgrass	Root	*Polygonum*
Madrone	Bark, leaves	*Arbutus*
Oak	Bark	*Quercus*
Persimmon	Green fruit, bark	*Diospyros*
Pigweed	Leaves	*Amaranthus*
Pine	Needles	*Pinus*
Plantain	Leaves, root	*Plantago*
Rattlesnake fern	Leaves	*Botrychium*
Redbud	Buds	*Cercis*
Sea-lavender	Root	*Limonium*

Spicebush	Bark	*Lindera*
Sumac	Roots	*Rhus*
Sunflower	Leaves	*Helianthus*
Wild azalea	Leaves, flowers, stems	*Rhododendron*
Wild indigo	Leaves, branches	*Baptisia*
Yarrow	Flowers	*Achillea*

ADDITIONAL READINGS

Askinson, George William.
    1922. *Perfumes and Cosmetics.* 392 pp. Norman W. Henley Pub-
    lishing Company, 2 West Forty-fifth Street, New York, New York
    10017.

Christiana, Richard S.
    1877. *Perfumery and Kindred Arts.* 386 pp. H. C. Baird and
    Company, Philadelphia, Pennsylvania.

    1915. *The Druggist' Circular Formula Book.* 3d ed. 242 pp., illus.
    The Druggist Circular. New York, New York.

Heelrick, U. P., editor
    1919. *Sturtevant's Notes on Edible Plants.* 686 pp. J. P. Lyon
    Company, State Printers, Albany, New York.

Hiss, A. Emil.
    1914. *Perfume and Toilet Articles.* 430 pp. G. P. Engelhard and
    Company, Chicago, Illinois.

Klebs, Arnold.
    1925. *Catalogue of Early Herbals.* 118 pp. L'Art Ancien S.A.,
    Lugano, Switzerland.

Koller, Theodore.
    1920. *Cosmetics.* 262 pp. Scott, Greenwood and Son, London,
    England.

Krochmal, Arnold, and Connie Krochmal.
    1973. *A Guide to Medicinal Plants of the United States.* 350 pp.,
    illus. Quadrangle/The New York Times Book Co., New York, New
    York.

Leyel, Mrs. C. F.
    1926. *The Magic of Herbs.* 320 pp. Jonathan Cape, Thirty Bed-
    ford Square, London, England.

Magness, J. R.; G. M. Markle; C. C. Compton.
1971. *Food and Field Crops of the United States.* 254 pp. Inter-regional Research Project IR-4, I. R. Bulletin No. 1, Rutgers University, New Brunswick, New Jersey 08901.

Martin, Geoffrey.
1921. *Perfumes, Essential Oils, and Fruit Essences.* 138 pp. C. Lockwood and Son, London, England.

Parry, Ernest J.
1925. *Parry's Cyclopedia of Perfumery.* 2 vols. 838 pp. P. Blakiston's Son and Company, Philadelphia, Pennsylvania.

Piesse, Charles H.
1891. *The Art of Perfumery.* 5th ed. 498 pp., illus. Piesse and Lubin, New Bedford Street, London, England.

Poucher, William Arthur.
1936. *Perfumes, Cosmetics and Soaps.* 2 vols. 866 pp., illus. Chapman and Hall Ltd., London, England.

Rohde, Eleanor Sinclair.
1922. *The Old English Herbals.* 243 pp., illus. Longmans, Green and Company, London, England.

Sagarin, Edward.
1945. *The Science and Art of Perfumery.* 268 pp., illus. McGraw-Hill, New York, New York.

Thompson, C. J. S.
1927. *The Mystery and Lure of Perfume.* 247 pp., illus. John Lane, The Bodley Head Ltd., London, England.

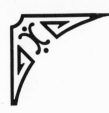
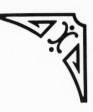

Index

73 74 75 5 4 3 2 1